NUTRITION

A PRACTICAL APPROACH
For
HOLISTIC THERAPISTS

SUZANNE REED-LE-QUESNE

HEALTH & BEAUTY ENTERPRISES

First Published in 2001
by Health & Beauty Enterprises

ISBN 0–9540520–0–5

Typeset, Printed and Bound by The Charlesworth Group, Huddersfield, UK.
01484 517077

ABOUT THE AUTHOR

With fourteen years experience in the health business Suzanne Reed-Le Quesne has become a leading authority on nutrition and holistic therapies and has established Holistic Training schools in the Channel Islands and the West Midlands.

Suzanne's primary role is as a Clinical Nutritionist. She graduated from the Institute of Optimum Nutrition, London in 1993 under the guidance of Patrick Holford, the founder of the Institute, who was her tutor in her final year. Suzanne now holds nutrition/allergy clinics, run seminars and workshops all over the UK and has also worked in Europe.

Suzanne's most recent personal training has been in the field of the psychology of eating disorders and is part of a team of specialists manning a phone-in help line for people suffering from disordered eating patterns.

Suzanne wrote the very popular Home Study Diploma course in Nutrition in 1998 accredited by Vocational Awards International which has been successfully completed by students all over the world.

Suzanne is a member of the British Association of Nutritional Therapists, the Association of Therapy Lecturers, a full member of the Guild of Health Writers, and founder member of the Jersey Association of Complementary Therapists, she was also a tutor at the Institute for Optimum Nutrition in London during 1995 and 1996.

In addition to her role as a nutrition consultant, she is also a leading authority on nutrition, and is an established speaker and broadcaster.

ACKNOWLEDGEMENTS

I would like to express my deepest gratitude to my husband Barry for all his help in the preparation of this book. His patience is second to none, and his assistance as a helpful listener, proofreader and endless time in cross-referencing the work has been irreplaceable. Without his continued support and encouragement this book would never have been completed.

Very special thanks also to many friends, colleagues, past and present students for their continual support, invaluable feedback, and input.

FOREWORD

With so many books published every year in the field of nutrition and herbal medicine, it is almost inconceivable to imagine an area that remains virtually untapped. Well, Suzanne Reed has done it! When I first heard about her book *Nutrition – A Practical Approach for Holistic Therapists* I became especially interested. This was, in part, because I knew that she would handle the subject with great care, knowledge and professionalism, but also because the audience that she was targeting has seldom, if ever, had nutrition books that were directed to their special requirements.

In recent times, complementary health practitioners in fields such as homeopathy, massotherapy, herbalism, aromatherapy, and many others have seen the value of incorporating nutrition in their practice. This book provides an excellent blueprint for such practitioners to use in order to augment their main form of therapy with both dietary manipulation and the use of prudent and safe supplementation. Equally students who wish to become practitioners of nutrition or other forms of natural medicine will find this a hugely valuable tool to complement their qualification course. And this is not only the case in terms of background in the therapeutic and preventative principle of nutrition. Suzanne also addresses the science of food, background in numerous common health disorders and the often-overlooked skills in pre- and post- care assessment and follow-up. In fact, this manual will also be a useful reference for those who are already qualified in the field of nutrition.

Suzanne is a multi-faceted and multi-qualified practitioner who has truly embraced the principle of 'holistic'. Her experience and understanding of the need to address the *whole* person is certainly reflected in *Nutrition – A Practical Approach for Holistic Therapists*. Holistic medicine *is* the future of healthcare, and this ambitious and much needed book will help complementary medicine practitioners and students to even more successfully empower people to achieve true health and wellness.

Stephen Terrass MRNT
February 2001

INTRODUCTION

This book has been written out of true need. Much of my time is spent teaching postgraduate courses in advanced holistic therapies. It never ceases to amaze me at how little knowledge therapists have regarding good nutrition and the little, if any, knowledge therapists have of the symptoms their clients present.

The general public is becoming more and more responsible for their own health. Unfortunately they are often bombarded with so much conflicting information they do not know which way to turn. More and more are turning to us, holistic and health practitioners for guidance and it is therefore our professional duty to keep learning beyond our initial basic training by way of Continued Personal Development in order to be of maximum help to our clients.

As holistic therapists you should always undertake a thorough client consultation before giving any treatment and whist many of you do, many do not, and others only record the barest minimum details due to restricted allocated time for treatments. The consultation is of course the essence to a successful treatment and is what puts us ahead of the General Practitioners who just do not have the time to talk with and listen to their patients. Those of you in a salon situation should encourage employers for additional consultation time for maximum client benefit.

Additionally as holistic therapists you should always offer relevant and specific after-care advice to each client. Again, whilst most of you do, others do not and, again, with tight appointment schedules, many therapist just do not have the time. It is of paramount importance to give individual after-care advice to make the treatment special and tailor-made for each client.

With the help of this book you will now be able to expand the consultation process by learning what important questions to ask clients regarding their nutritional status and nutritional deficiencies/ excesses that may be responsible for the symptoms they present. You will have a clearer understanding of those symptoms and as such you will be able to use this book as an instant reference guide for tailor-made responsible after-care advice.

The after-care recommendations are listed by way of the very latest and safest supernutrients, vitamin and mineral supplements, herbal remedies, superfoods, lifestyle changes and of course dietary advice.

I am a firm believer in the holistic approach treating mind, body and spirit as one. I also believe that by establishing the weakest link, that is the weakest body system, and then supporting that system by way of holistic treatments, dietary supplements and diet, the result will be a domino effect on the other body systems that will eventually make the body whole and strong again.

Long term effects of poor diet and nutrition are given for each body system. The digestive and excretory systems are the largest and most detailed chapters and are covered in greater detail to cover the underpinning knowledge required by many awarding bodies offering nutritional qualifications.

The Weakest Link questionnaire is a quick and easy way to establish your clients weakest body system, for which you can then offer support. You can then build on this initial questionnaire to establish your client's current diet and integrate the whole into your own client consultation form.

Our aim as holistic therapists is to educate, enlighten, encourage and help our clients help themselves on the way to good health.

It would have been an impossible task to record every symptom a client will ever present to you. I have included therefore the most frequently encountered symptoms I come across in my role as clinical nutritionist, presented system by system. There are over 100 of the most common ailments listed and recommendations for each of them, as well as recommendations for the system in general.

All our food ultimately comes from plants, and second hand from animals who eat the plants, and our daily intake of food should supply us with all the nutrients needed to sustain health and vitality.

Unfortunately, with the ever increasing use of ready-made and fast foods many people are not receiving all the nutrients they need from food and many can be said to be overfed but undernourished.

Even fresh organic food may be nutrient deficient. It may be void of pesticides but may still grown in nutrient deficient soil.

As a nation we are consuming fewer calories in an effort to reduce weight but getting fatter. The cravings many experience are not cravings for more food but cravings for more nutrients hence we are eating more and more and going around in ever increasing circles.

Unfortunately the result of years of being undernourished but over fed are many diseases, which can be directly linked to diet. 90% of the world's cancers are diet related and as such are preventable.

The time has come to take action. We must help ourselves and our clients find the weakest link in our health by studying each body system in turn and then do everything we can to support that system. A domino effect may then happen, strengthening each body system in turn and bringing the body back to a healthy whole.

There are 42 nutrients known to be of importance to man, the most abundant being the macronutrients, the carbohydrates, fats, and proteins, and the micro-nutrients the vitamins, minerals, trace minerals, fresh clean water and fresh clean air. We need all of them daily for maximum health.

REMEMBER
PRACTISE WHAT YOU PREACH!

HOW TO USE THIS BOOK

This book may appear long and complex. However, it is very easy to use.

The Weakest Link questionnaire given in Part III will only take a few minutes of your client's time but when completed you will be able to see at a glance the client's weakest link. That is, the system of the body which needs the most support at the time of the consultation and treatment for that day.

Therefore, by adding the results of the Weakest Link questionnaire to your usual client consultation you will know what system of the body is in need of most dietary, supplement or other support.

Once you have established the client's weakest body system by using the Weakest Link Questionnaire, refer to the relevant chapter and read the general recommendations given for that system. If your client's particular symptom is listed, then refer directly to that symptom, as well as the general recommendations. Discuss the recommendations with the client and choose one or two the client can commit to. These may be changes in diet to either include or avoid a particular food or drink, or it may be to take a herbal or vitamin supplement, or to start eating a superfood or to adopt a lifestyle change. By discussing the recommendations and getting the client's approval of what they feel they can take on board, you are far more likely to get good results with that client.

The after-care advice you give your client will then truly become 'tailor made' for every treatment you undertake. Whilst 'drink more water, rest and eat a light diet' will of course always be essential and excellent after care advice, as holistic therapists you need to expand on your after care and recommend specific support to each client.

If you enjoy using the Weakest Link questionnaire you can take it further by making up for yourself a more detailed Nutritional Questionnaire to accompany your own consultation. This will give you even more information and you can then expand your treatments to always include some nutritional recommendations. Alternatively you may wish to give separate consultations just for nutrition alone in which case taking a formal qualification is highly recommended.

AUTHOR'S NOTE

In my role as Clinical Nutritionist I see many hundreds of clients a year and nothing gives me more pleasure than seeing their health improve.

There may be times when you want to recommend more than one supplement in an attempt to achieve the most beneficial result for your client. However, unless you are qualified to do so, please do not be tempted to do this. Whilst nutritional supplements are generally safe, offering a cocktail of individual supplements requires training. Excesses of some nutrients may result in deficiencies of others. Multivitamin and mineral formulas are therefore always a safe choice as experienced nutritionists have correctly formulated their content.

Please therefore only offer one recommendation by way of food supplement or herbal supplement and ask the client to use this for three to four months. If there is no improvement then you can go on to another of the food supplements or herbal supplement recommendations. Always emphasise to the client to follow the manufacturer's instructions on the label when recommending any supplement.

It is perfectly safe to offer dietary advice in conjunction with a nutritional supplement, in fact the two go hand in hand.

Foods and supplements should not be relied upon alone to treat or prevent disease and should never replace medication without consulting your GP.

Never treat outside your own knowledge and never be ashamed or embarrassed to refer a client to someone more experienced than yourself in a particular field.

Do not expect all foods and supplements to work the same way on all people, we are all bio-chemically different and therefore all have different needs.

No single food or food type should ever be eaten to the exclusion of others for the purposes of preventing or addressing a specific disease or maintaining health except on the advise of a GP.

Suzanne Reed-Le Quesne
February, 2001

CONTENTS

PART II   Body Systems

Part III – Putting it all together

SELF-TEST PAPERS   WHAT HAVE YOU REMEMBERED?

PART 1   THE BASICS

NUTRIENTS

Nutrients — What exactly are they?

They are absorbable components of food. The six important nutrients are carbohydrates, proteins, fats, minerals, vitamins and water.

Main functions

Necessary for good health, energy, organ function, food utilisation and cell growth.

What do nutrients actually do?

Nutrients maintain life. The macronutrients, the carbohydrates, fats and proteins provide energy and the micronutrients, the vitamins and minerals are the substances required to release the energy. The amounts of macronutrients and micronutrients needed daily to maintain life is enormously different but each vitally important.

CARBOHYDRATES

Carbohydrates – What exactly are they?

Carbohydrates are composed of oxygen, hydrogen and carbon.

Main function

Carbohydrates are our primary source of energy.

What exactly do carbohydrates do?

Carbohydrates are the main source of energy for all body functions and muscular exertion. The term carbohydrate includes a variety of dietary compounds varying from simple sugars at the one end to complex structures composed of many interlinked sugar molecules at the other. Simple carbohydrates are referred to as sugars. A single sugar is known as a mono-saccharide. When two sugar molecules are joined together they become a di-saccharide, and when many di-saccharides are joined together they become polysaccharides. A polysaccharide is therefore composed of several chains of single sugars interlinked with one another. It is the polysaccharides that are referred to as complex carbohydrates.

Simple sugars such as those in fruit and honey are very easily digested. Double sugars such as sucrose (table sugar), require some digestive action, but the polysaccharides require prolonged enzymatic action in order to be broken down into simple sugars ready for absorption.

An example of a simple carbohydrate is glucose. The ending "ose" indicates that it is a sugar. Glucose is therefore a mono-saccharide.

The main difference between them is that the mono-saccarides and the di-saccarides are water-soluble. This means they are readily absorbed into the body through the stomach giving a burst of energy. The complex variety, the polysaccharides, on the other hand, need digesting through the small intestine, and therefore give a more steady energy burst for a longer period of time.

It is the complex carbohydrates or the polysaccharides that are needed for sustained energy and to keep blood glucose levels steady.

The most important carbohydrate is glucose, a mono-saccharide that circulates in our blood to supply energy to cells throughout the body. It is used as an energy source by all other living things as well. The body's metabolism and energy systems have a high demand for glucose. For example, it is the only source of energy usable by the brain, and a low level of glucose in the blood results in a disturbance in brain function such as loss of concentration, even to the point of coma. When a doctor measures your blood sugar level, he is actually measuring your blood glucose level at that particular time. To have a good indication of your blood sugar status you would require a six-hour glucose test, which would measure the body's response to glucose over that time. (*see Appendix 1*)

In our modern diet, polysaccharides should comprise about 50 per cent of carbohydrate intake. However, it is estimated that sucrose (glucose and fructose combined to make ordinary table sugar) comprises about 30 per cent of carbohydrate intake, lactose (milk sugar) comprises about 10 per cent, and other less important sugars form the remaining 10 per cent. Historically, our ancestors consumed considerably more complex carbohydrate, and it is only since the middle of the nineteenth century that our intake of refined carbohydrates, particularly sucrose, has been significant, resulting in higher numbers of people who have difficulty in maintaining an even blood sugar level.

The metabolism of carbohydrates is geared to the digestion of complex carbohydrates in the gastrointestinal tract. Digestive enzymes in saliva and pancreatic secretions break down complex polysaccharides into their component mono and di-saccharides. The di-sacchariades are further digested by enzymes present in the lining of the small intestine. In this way, all sugars are broken down to mono-saccharides which are then easily absorbed into the bloodstream, from which they pass to the liver.

THE SUGAR FAMILY

At the top of the tree come the quickly digested mono-saccharide sugars like glucose and fructose – fruit and corn.

Then comes the di-saccharide sugars, sucrose, dextrose, maltose and lactose coming in foods like white and brown sugar, overcooked grains, honey and milk products.

And lastly, the polysaccharides, the slow releasing carbohydrates, like grains, lentils, beans, potatoes and vegetables.

We can also add to the bottom of this family tree the indigestible polysaccharides otherwise known as fibre, which can also be found in grains, lentils, beans, carbohydrates and vegetables.

SIMPLE SUGARS	GLUCOSE (blood sugar)	fruits, corn.
	FRUCTOSE (fruit sugar)	berries and grapes
	SUCROSE (table sugar)	white & brown sugar
	DEXTROSE	overcooked grains
	MALTOSE	honey
	LACTOSE (milk sugar)	milk products
COMPLEX CARBOHYDRATES	POLYSACCHARIDES (or starches)	grains, lentils, beans, potatoes vegetables
	INDIGESTIBLE POLYSACCHARIDES (cellulose or fibre)	The fibre in grains lentils, vegetables beans

WHICH FORMS OF SUGAR ARE BEST?

Any food containing complex carbohydrate, or naturally rich in fructose and vitamins or minerals is far better than refined sugar, honey or malt. That means beans, lentils, seeds, grains and vegetables (provided they're not overcooked), as well as fresh fruit are all good 'complex' sources of sugar.

Provided you avoid all forms of refined sugar, and don't have too much concentrated natural sugar as in pure juice (which should always be diluted with water) or dried fruit, there is no reason to be concerned about how much sugar your diet provides.

FIBRE

Fibre can be classified as soluble or insoluble but both are largely indigestible by human beings, but important in our diets for different reasons. They are only found in plant foods.

Soluble fibre is soluble in water and include pectins found in apples and gums found in beans, some fruits, vegetables, oats, and barley. Soluble fibre takes up bile acids, cholesterol and toxins and carries them out of the body. They therefore lower harmful cholesterol levels and reduce the risk of cardiovascular disease. Soluble fibre absorbs many times its volume of water, soothes the intestinal tract, eases bowel movements by making stools slippery and also provides food for beneficial bacteria in the intestines.

Insoluble fibre is not soluble in water. It helps against weight gain, colon cancer and gallstones. However an excess of insoluble fibre can irritate the delicate lining of the intestinal tract. Insoluble fibre such as wheat bran is a harsher type of fibre and adds bulk to our stools. By bulking the waste, it can move more rapidly through the system thus preventing constipation. It also helps against irritable bowel syndrome, haemorrhoids, diverticulosis, varicose veins and cancer of the colon. Cellulose and hemicellulose are other kinds of harsher insoluble fibre and can be found in foods such as whole-wheat flour, bran, cabbage, green beans, and broccoli.

REMEMBER
If you cook complex carbohydrates too long they change their molecular structure and become a 'simple' carbohydrate – don't overcook food.

HOW MUCH FIBRE DO YOU NEED?

The average adult needs to eat no less than 35 g. of fibre per day. The best way is to eat fibre is where it occurs naturally – for instance, in starchy foods, vegetables and fruits.

The ideas below will provide approximately 18 g of figre. The remainder will come from your 5 daily portions of vegetables and fruit.

Ideas to meet your daily fibre needs:-
2 Shredded Wheat, a medium portion of wholemeal pasta, an orange and a generous serving of broccoli.

or

2 digestive biscuits. a medium portion of baked beans with 2 slices of wholemeal toast

or

A bowl of All-Bran and three dried apricots

or

2 Weetabix, a slice of wholemeal toast, a small packet of nuts and a medium portion of brown rice risotto.

Eating enough fibre may also help guard against breast cancer, either directly or indirectly. Women who eat more vegetables and fruit and starchy wholegrain cereals have a lower incidence of breast cancer, whereas a high intake of red meat and fried or browned food may increase the risk.

CARBOHYDRATE LOADING BEFORE AND AFTER SPORT.

Athletes are big fans of starchy food. Most elite athletes eat a high-carbohydrate diet for a few days before an endurance event. This is called carbohydrate loading. They also eat a starchy pre-event meal, to boost their energy and endurance. The body turns the starches into glucose and glycogen, to provide both instant and stored energy for the brain and muscles. Starches are a better source of energy than sugar because they contain more nutrients and fibre.

Most of us don't need to eat the massive quantities of carbohydrates consumed by top athletes. We can however, all benefit from a little carbohydrate loading after exercise, when a starchy snack (as opposed to sugary confectionery, fizzy drinks or fatty food) is a better way of replenishing depleted energy. A banana and some water is lot less expensive than a fashionable sports drink – and does the job of re-hydrating and boosting energy very efficiently.

VEGETABLES AND FRUIT – AT LEAST 5 PORTIONS A DAY

Fruit is the ultimate convenience food, requiring little or no prepara-tion. It is easy to carry and enjoyable to eat any time, anywhere, making it a versatile snack. Vegetables are an integral part of all healthy meals. For optimum nutrition, five portions of vegetables and fruit per day are highly recommended —and there is probably even more benefit in consuming more, if you want to. Because most fruit can be eaten raw, and many vegetables can be eaten raw in salads, or lightly cooked, they retain all their vitamins and minerals (when eaten fresh), which in other foods are depleted or destroyed by cooking. Vegetables and fruit include all fresh, frozen, chilled and canned varieties (with the exception of potatoes, which are a starchy food). Also included are dried fruits and fruit juices, but not fruit flavoured drinks which contain very little, if any, fruit juice and a lot of added sugars or sweeteners and other non-nutritious ingredients.

ENZYMES & DIGESTIVE ENZYMES

Enzymes – What exactly are they?

Enzymes are a delicate lifelike substance found in all living cells whether animal or vegetable. Enzymes are energised protein molecules that perform specific biochemical reactions vital for life. They are protein catalysts.

Main functions

There are three classes of enzymes. Digestive, metabolic and food. The main function of digestive enzymes are to break down food into particles chemically simple enough and physically small enough to be absorbed. The main function of metabolic enzymes are to carry out millions of chemical activities in our bodies every second to keep us alive and the main function of food enzymes are to start food digestion.

What exactly do enzymes do?

Enzymes change one substance to another, without actually changing themselves. Digestive enzymes break down the food we eat into substances that can be absorbed. There are three types of digestive enzyme. Amylases, which digest carbohydrate, proteases which digest protein and lipases which digest fat.

All the organs and tissue in our bodies are run by metabolic enzymes. These enzyme workers take amino acids, fatty acids, and simple sugars and structure them into healthy bodies, keeping everything working properly. Every organ and tissue has its own particular metabolic enzymes that do specialised work.

Food enzymes from raw food contain natural enzymes that cooking destroys. When raw food enters the mouth, and the food is chewed well, their natural enzymes start to breakdown the food as a natural digestive process. These natural enzymes are not destroyed by stomach acid but are active throughout the digestive tract, right through to the large colon where they create good conditions for beneficial bacteria to grow.

Many of these digestive and metabolic enzymes are dependent upon vitamins and minerals to activate them. Enzymes are made up of two parts, one is a protein molecule and the other is a coenzyme. The coenzyme is often a vitamin, a mineral or both. So if you are nutrient deficient, you will not make the enzymes necessary to carry out their important work. For example, zinc is needed to make hydrochloric acid (stomach acid) and protease (a protein splitting enzyme). If a person becomes deficient in the mineral zinc, their production of stomach acid will decline and they will have difficulty in breaking down protein. This can then lead on to other problems further down the digestive tract.

Our bodies produce 25% of the enzymes we need for digestion, the other 75% is expected to come from natural, raw, unprocessed sources in our fruit, vegetables, grains and nuts. Many people have difficulty in eating 5 portions of fruit and vegetables every day, so you can see how quickly the body may become deficient and overtax the body's pancreas and other enzymes. This often results in indigestion, heartburn and fatigue. By eating raw, or lightly cooked vegetables and fruit you are providing natural enzymes to assist in breaking down all the food eaten at one meal, at the same time providing essential nutrients (coenzymes) to activate other metabolic enzymes to keep the body working efficiently. These natural enzymes cannot be stored in the body, so fresh vegetables and fruit should be eaten with every meal.

EXAMPLES OF FOODS THAT CONTAIN SIGNIFICANT AMOUNTS OF ENZYMES

Apples and mangos contain peroxidase and catalase whose job it is to disarm free radicals.
Pineapple, wheat and kidney beans contain amylase, which digests sugars and protease which digests protein.
Mushrooms contain amylase, protease, peroxidase and catalase.
Bananas and cabbage contain amylase.
Raw eggs contain the four enzymes already mentioned and lipase.

This is not a complete list and there are many more foods being investigated.

Nutritionists often recommend digestive enzymes to aid digestion and nutrient absorption. Many consider insufficient digestive enzymes, of which stress plays a big part, is the cause of many digestive system complains. Vegetarians and vegans should read labels carefully as some digestive enzymes contain ox bile extract. There are several companies who manufacture vegetarian and vegan digestive enzymes. These digestive enzymes are often used as a temporary measure, but the long term answer is to eat fresh, natural fruits and vegetables on a daily basis.

REMEMBER

Fruits and Vegetables contain vitamins and minerals
and are vital for 'enzyme action'

5 portions a day, every day, are highly recommended

PROTEINS

Proteins – What exactly are they?

Proteins are composed of oxygen, hydrogen, carbon and nitrogen.

Main function

For the growth and repair of body tissues and production of enzymes.

What do proteins actually do?

The Greek meaning of protein is 'of prime importance', and after water, is the most plentiful substance in the body. Proteins are also the most complex of all food compounds, the key factor of protein is nitrogen, the crucial ingredient in the formation of amino and nucleic acids (both nitrogen-containing compounds).

Without protein we would be unable to rebuild body cells, tissue, muscles and organs and synthesise many important enzymes, neuro-transmitters (used in the nervous system like seratonin), the important structural proteins that make hair and nails, and the all important hormones of the endocrine system. However many people have put too much importance on protein and as a result we tend to eat excess which may be an important factor or precursor in many modern diseases, including osteoporosis, water retention and acidity.

Proteins are macronutrients that are supplied in the diet, digested to amino acids and absorbed in the gastrointestinal tract to be rebuilt by the body into its own proteins. To maintain good health there are eight 'essential' amino acids that human beings must have every day. The body is unable to synthesise these amino acids and so we must actually ingest them on a daily basis. It is thought that we used to be able to synthesize these essential amino acids but somehow lost the ability to do so along the path of evolution.

When we think of protein foods, we tend to think immediately of meat, poultry, fish, eggs and cheese and, indeed about 30 years ago these protein foods were called 'first class protein' as they contain all the 'essential' amino acids needed for human growth and health.

Nuts, peas, beans and lentils used to be called 'second class proteins' as although they contain all the essential amino acids, they appear in smaller quantities and some of these more vegetarian types of foods may be low in one particular amino acid. It was therefore felt that they were only 'second class'.

Fortunately, these labels have been dropped and replaced with 'complete' protein foods and 'incomplete' protein foods that have a 'limiting' amino acid — which is somewhat a better description.

A limiting amino acid is an amino acid that is present in relatively small amounts and below the recommended essential amino acid requirements. Examples would be quinoa and wheat, both of which are short in the amino acid lysine. Lysine would therefore be called the limiting amino acid. A vegetarian would therefore have to 'top up' with lysine by taking a supplement or by eating foods high in lysine, which would include soybeans, pinto beans and other legumes. These foods would then be called complementary foods.

A complete protein is therefore any food substance that contains all 8 Essential Amino Acids. Eggs are an excellent example of a complete protein, with all its essential amino acids in the correct proportions. Other complete protein foods are fish, meat, and cheese.

An egg is therefore probably the best food we can eat for our complete daily requirement of protein. However, the egg must be boiled, poached or baked for full benefit. Eggs contain a substance called lecithin, which is also a component of bile. The function of lecithin is to break down fat. If we fry eggs the high temperature destroys the lecithin and therefore fried eggs become a high cholesterol food. However, when boiled, poached or baked, the lecithin remains in tact and the cholesterol is used as nature intended — to break down and utilise the cholesterol in the egg.

REMEMBER
The protein in an egg is found in the whites
the yolk contains the harmful saturated fat

VEGETARIANS

Vegetarians need to be careful in selecting their food intake in order to consume complete protein meals. Protein is found in all foods and is especially high in complex carbohydrate foods such as quinoa (a grain particularly high in protein) peas, beans, lentils, and rice.

By eating a combination of various foods (not necessarily at one meal – as the body has an 'amino acid pool' that can provide a 48 hour supply) then the vegetarian can be sure of ingesting enough of all the 8 essential amino acids for their needs.

30gms of rice, for example, contains 21gms of complete protein and 30gms of broad beans provides 14gms of complete protein so by eating both you will get 28gms of protein in the right proportions (almost the equivalent of one egg that provides 30gms of complete protein).

Vegetarians do not have difficulty in obtaining enough protein and there are many studies to suggest vegetarians are healthier than meat/

poultry eaters, with less risk of cardiovascular disease, cancer and diabetes.

THE ESSENTIAL AMINO ACIDS

There are 26 known amino acids and as mentioned earlier 8 of these are known as 'essential'.

Essential Amino Acids

Arginine (in children) and Histidine (in children)
Isoleucine, Leucine, Lysine, Methionine
Phenylalanine, Threonine, Tryptophan, Valine

The body has an 'amino acid pool' where amino acids are stored until required. From the 8 essential amino acids the others can be synthesized by a method called transamination which takes place in the liver. Synthesis by the body requires vitamin A. High protein intakes require concomitant vitamin A intake. Vitamin B6 (pyridoxine) is also required for protein synthesis.

The liver needs particular nutrients to convert and rebuild amino acids. Vitamins A, B6, as mentioned above, together with vitamin K and B12 are the important nutrients needed for this function.

SOME IMPORTANT FUNCTIONS OF THE 8 ESSENTIAL AMINO ACIDS

ARGININE (an essential amino acid in children)
♦ Accelerates wound healing.
♦ Stimulates human growth hormone (HGH) which stimulates immune function.
♦ Necessary for normal sperm count.
♦ Enhances fat metabolism.
♦ Involved in insulin production.

HISTIDINE (an essential amino acid in children)
♦ Helps to remove toxic metals from the body.
♦ Effective in treating ulcers in the digestive tract.

- Has been successfully used in the treatment of rheumatoid arthritis.
- Helps maintain the myelin sheaths which insulate the nerves and is required by the auditory nerve for good function.
- Stimulates the production of red and white blood cells.

LEUCINE and ISOLEUCINE
- Two of the amino acids know as the Branched Chain Amino Acids.
- Both are commonly deficient in amino acid profiles of chronically sick individuals.
- Isoleucine is useful in formation of haemoglobin.

LYSINE
- Often low in vegetarian diets.
- Important in children's growth and development.
- Helps in the formation of antibodies to fight disease.
- Effective in treatment of herpes simplex virus, especially when combined with Vitamin C.
- Enhances concentration.

METHIONINE
- An essential amino acid containing sulphur.
- A powerful antioxidant preventing free radical damage to body tissues.
- Acts to detoxify heavy metals from the body.
- Strengthens hair follicles
- Assists gallbladder function through synthesis of bile salts.

PHENYLALANINE
- Required by the thyroid for normal function.
- Needs Vitamin C to be metabolised.
- Acts as an anti-depressant.
- May improve memory, concentration and mental alertness.

THREONINE
- Prevents accumulation of fat in the liver.
- Required for digestive and intestinal tract function.

◆ Deficient in grains, but abundant in pulses, making a combination of grains and pulses a complete source of protein for vegetarians (beans on toast for example).
◆ Suggested being essential for mental health.

TRYPTOPHAN
◆ Needed for the synthesis of Vitamin B3 in the body and the precursor of the neurotransmitter serotonin, which is a calming, sedating substance essential for normal mood and sleep patterns.
◆ Has powerful painkilling effects.
◆ Useful in weight control.
◆ Acts as a mood adaptogen – calms agitation, stimulates depressed individuals).

VALINE
◆ Needed for normalising the nitrogen balance in the body.
◆ Vital for mental function, in muscle coordination and neural function.
◆ Helpful in cases of inflammation.
◆ A branched-chain amino acid.

BRANCHED CHAIN AMINO ACIDS
The branch chain amino acids, valine, leucine and isoleucine – protect all muscles, including the heart, and actually makes exercise seem more enjoyable by reducing the feeling of fatigue.

HOW MUCH PROTEIN DO YOU ACTUALLY NEED?
Children need more protein than adults. Most nutritionists agree that after the age of 19 protein requirements stop increasing and remain at approximately 2ozs per day (55g) for a medium sized man and 1½ozs (45g) per day for a medium sized woman. So whilst vitally important to our diet, we do not need very much of it — approximately 15% of our total daily calorie intake. So if you were consuming 2000 calories per day, your protein requirement would be approximately 300 calories. Choose low fat protein sources like turkey, chicken, cottage cheese, fish and tofu.

It is quite difficult to become protein deficient in the Western world. However, there are instances, particularly in the case of inexperienced vegetarians, vegans, or people on calorie restricting diets not to get enough. Protein deficiency can be a cause of fluid retention in the body and abnormalities of growth and tissue development. The hair, nails and skin specially will be affected, and muscle tone will be poor.

FATS

Fats – What exactly are they?

Fats are composed of oxygen, hydrogen and carbon.

Main functions

Fats provide a highly concentrated source of energy, which can be stored and used instead of carbohydrates when necessary. Fats provide us with insulation and protect delicate body organs. Fats also produce highly active biological substances that are vital for the normal working of the body. These substances are known as prostaglandins.

Fats – What exactly do fats do?

Out of all the macronutrients, fats are often the most misunderstood. As with the other macronutrients, fats can also be divided into groups. The main three groups are:

**Saturated fats
Mono-unsaturated fats
Poly-unsaturated fats.**

Saturated fats are the most damaging to health. They clog up the arteries and are one of the main causes of obesity, which itself brings a host of other health problems, and are recognised to be a factor in hypertension and heart disease. Saturated fats are hard at room temperature like butter, margarine and lard. Saturated fats are responsible for inflammatory actions in the body. There are many other 'hidden' fats in foods like biscuits, cakes and all confectionery.

> ## REMEMBER
> Saturated fats are hard at room temperature. If a 'healthy' margarine is advertised as poly-unsaturated – but is hard at room temperature then it is a saturated fat.
> It was poly-unsaturated at one time but food processing has made it 'saturated'.

Mono-Unsaturated fats are the fats that should be used in cooking. As a result of their chemical make-up they remain stable at high temperatures. The best oil for this purpose is cold pressed Virgin Olive Oil. It is good for us, as it is unrefined and therefore more beneficial than the refined vegetable oils like sunflower oil available in supermarkets.

Pistachio nuts are one of the highest nuts in content of monounsaturated fats, coming in at 67%. In general, nuts have a higher polyunsaturated:saturated fatty acid ratio and a higher amount of monounsaturated fats. Studies with walnuts and almonds have shown benefit in lowering total cholesterol and other cardiovascular risk factors. Many people have steered away from consuming nuts due to their high fat and calorie content with concerns that this would increase cardiovascular risk. This has not been shown to be the case. As long as one is not sensitive to a particular nut, I encourage consumption of nuts not only because of their essential fatty acid content but also their fibre and vitamin E content as an alternative to saturated fats or animal protein.

Polyunsaturated fats – these fats are 'liquid' at room temperature. Any oils that come in bottles like walnut, corn and sesame are classed as polyunsaturated. These oils should not be used for cooking but for salad dressings, or to put on vegetables instead of a saturated fat like butter. Poly-unsaturated fats are responsible for anti-inflammatory actions in the body.

As natural anti-inflammatories these polyunsaturated fats are essential in the maintenance of eczema, allergies, asthma, arthritis and many other inflammatory response in the body.

The poly-unsaturated fats can also be described as Essential Fatty Acids. As with the essential amino acids, the word 'essential' here means that human beings cannot synthesise fatty acids in the body and these substances must therefore be ingested every day as food.

Unfortunately, because of the mass production of food and the ever-increasing amounts of 'convenience' foods our population eat, many people are deficient in essential fatty acids.

Another reason many people are deficient in essential fatty acids is that these foods are usually high in calories and as such have been 'doomed' by the 'weight-loss' industry. Avocados for example are a highly nutritious food, high in essential fatty acids, vitamins and minerals but because of their high calorie value, many people on calorie restricted diets will not eat them. Nuts too have received the same fate – high in essential fatty acids but also high in calories – but an excellent health food source of protein.

The polyunsaturated fatty acids can also be divided into two groups.

Ω 6 Fatty Acids

Ω 3 Fatty Acids

The Omega 6 group of fatty acids

We obtain the omega 6 group of essential fatty acids from the food we eat by way of linoleic acid which are found exclusively from seeds and their oils. We then convert this linoleic acid to GLA – gamma linolenic acid, which you are probably familiar with if you take Evening Primrose Oil. This in turn is converted to DGLA – di-homo gamma linolenic acid, and from there to substances called prostaglandins. Prostaglandins are hormone like substances which are very short lived and have important functions in the body They help keep the blood thin, they have anti-inflammatory influences on the joints, they prevent fluid retention, they help lower blood pressure and help insulin work efficiently.

Many people are deficient in the omega 6 group of fatty acids. Many, women in particular, shy away from any type of oil or fat because of the calorie content, in the misbelieve that all fats are bad, resulting in a deficiency state.

Even if we consumed enough seeds and their oils, there are many obstacles hindering the conversation from the original LA (linoleic acid) to GLA (gamma linolenic acid). These include smoking, drinking alcohol, and stress in its many forms (chemical, emotional, physical, mental). Consequently, without the GLA we cannot go on to make the DGLA or the all-important prostaglandings.

Omega 6 deficiency signs are high blood pressure, inflammatory problems like arthritis, difficulty in losing weight, dry eyes and skin including eczema. Good sources of the Omega 6 essential fatty acids are hemp, pumpkin, sunflower, safflower, sesame, corn, walnut, soya bean and wheatgerm oil where as much as 50 per cent of the fats in these oils comes from the Omega 6 family.

An excellent way of including these vital nutrients into your diet is by grinding the seeds in a coffee grinder. Two tablespoons per day sprinkled onto either cereal or over salads is considered an optimal intake. Alternatively two tablespoons of oil, sprinkled over lightly cooked vegetables or over salads would be just as effective.

The Omega 3 group of fatty acids.

We obtain the omega 3 group of essential fatty acids from the food we eat by way of linolenic acid found in oily fish. We convert this linolenic acid to two substances known as EPA (eicosaopentonic acid) and DHA (docosahexaenoic acid) and from there again to substances called prostaglandins.

Whereas with the omega 6 group of fats the prostaglandins are known as Series 1, with the omega 3 group they are known as Series 3 prostaglandins.

Omega 3 deficiency signs are dry skin, poor coordination and impaired vision, high blood pressure, inflammatory health problems, prone to infections and fluid retention.

Still short lived hormone like substances but with different functions in the body, the Series 3 prostaglandins are essential for proper brain function, coordination and mood, reducing the stickiness of the blood, controlling blood cholesterol and fat levels, improving immune function and metabolism, reducing inflammation and maintaining water balance.

An excellent way of including these vital nutrients into your diet is by eating oily fish like herring, salmon, sardines, and tuna at least 3 – 5 times each week. By eating oily fish you are bypassing the first conversion stage and taking into your diet directly the EPA and DHA. The best seed oils for the omega 3 group of fats are flax (also known as linseed), hemp and pumpkin.

Recommendation — In my practice I have no time to explain thoroughly to clients everything about fats, so I recommend a way of meeting the needs for both Omega 3 and Omega 6 fats in a way that is quick and easy. This is a product called Essential Balance *(Appendix I)* and just one tablespoon per day will meet all the necessary requirements of the Essential Fatty Acids.

As part of a balanced diet, the maximum you should be consuming in fats is 30%. 25% would be even more beneficial and the 5% would be deducted from the Saturated Fats column. This can be broken down as shown in the following table. The example is for somebody consuming 2000 calories per day.

RECOMMENDATIONS FOR FAT INTAKE		
10%Saturated Fats Non -Essential	Butter, Lard, Margarine Any fat hard at room temperature	200 Calories
10%Mono-unsaturated fats. Non-Essential	Olive Oil for cooking or for making salad dressings	200 Calories
10%Poly-unsaturated fats ESSENTIAL	Seeds, Seed Oils, oily fish Essential Balance	200 Calories

CHOLESTEROL

What exactly is it?

Cholesterol is a hard, waxy fatty substance that is essential for physical health, even though it is not required in our food supply, since our bodies can manufacture it.

Main functions

Cholesterol has four essential functions in the body.
◆ It is a constituent of cell membranes.
◆ It is a precursor of bile acids.
◆ It is a precursor of steroid hormones.
◆ Vitamin D, the sunshine vitamin, also comes from cholesterol.

What exactly does Cholesterol do?

As a constituent of cell membranes, cholesterol has the function of compensating for changes in membrane fluidity, keeping it within very narrow limits. This is such an important function that nature has equipped each cell with the means to synthesise its own membrane cholesterol. If cell membranes have too little cholesterol, they become too fluid and fall apart, if there is too much cholesterol they become stiff and break. The content of fatty acids in the diet varies from day to day and these fatty acids are used to build the basic structure of cell membranes. The more highly unsaturated fatty acids make membranes more fluid and the more saturated ones make them harder. The function of keeping the membranes within these light limits is a vital one.

The body makes 80% of the cholesterol it needs so there is no need to add cholesterol in the form of saturated animal fats from the diet.

Cholesterol is a precursor of bile acids and a main constituent of bile. Bile, produced in the liver and stored by the gallbladder, emulsifies (breaks down) fats into smaller globules ready for absorption. The absorption of fats, oils and fat-soluble vitamins could not be broken down and efficiently absorbed without bile.

Cholesterol is a precursor of steroid hormones. The female hormones oestrogen and progesterone and the male hormone testosterone are made from cholesterol.

Vitamin D the sunshine vitamin, required for the metabolism of calcium and phosphorus, also comes from cholesterol.

There are two types of cholesterol, harmful cholesterol known as LDLs (low density lipoproteins) and beneficial cholesterol known as HDLs (high density lipoproteins). Diet and exercise can play an important role in the levels of both these types of cholesterol.

Cholesterol exists in the blood and organs as HDL and LDL cholesterol. A high ratio of HDL to LDL is desirable to protect against atherosclerosis, arteriosclerosis and cardiovascular disease. Increasing the intake of polyunsaturated EFAs in favour of the harmful saturated animal fats can increase HDL.

Exercise is vital in reducing high levels of the harmful LDL cholesterol and increasing the HDLs. It is important for you to explain to your clients the benefits of exercise and that just one 30-minute gentle walk every day could make all the difference.

Many foods can assist in reducing high harmful cholesterol levels and preventing them becoming high in the first place. Regular daily fibre in the diet like fruit and vegetables and complex carbohydrates, will help remove the harmful LDL cholesterol. Apples, and other foods high in the soluble fibre pectin, can also reduce high cholesterol levels. In one French study a group of middle aged healthy men and women added two or three apples daily for a month to their diet. LDLs, the harmful cholesterol, fell in 80% of the group and by more than 10% in half of them, and beneficial HDLs increased. The study also showed better results on the women with one women's cholesterol being lowered by 30%.

Vitamin C, Vitamin E and other antioxidants can be described as anti-cholesterol supernutrients. They earn this title by the fact they destroy harmful free radicals that would otherwise turn the harmful LDL cholesterol toxic and even more dangerous. The antioxidants block free radicals and make LDL unable to infiltrate artery walls. Strawberries, guava, red peppers are high in Vitamin C. Sunflower seeds, walnuts, almonds, wheat germ, and soy beans high in Vitamin E, or an antioxidant supplement will give you protection.

TRIGLYCERIDES

What exactly are they?

Triglycerides are the main class of food fats. They make up about 95% of all the fats we eat as well as most of the stored fat we carry around in our bodies. They are a major way of storing energy for future use.

Main functions

Storage.
Protection.
Insulation.
Reserve for Essential Fatty Acids.
Conversion of sugars to fats.

What exactly do triglycerides do?

Storage — we store triglycerides as adipose tissue and this is used as a reserve of energy to be called upon in-between meals, while asleep, during increased exertion, during pregnancy or during famine.

Protection — the adipose tissue (stored triglycerides) also acts as a shock absorber to protect the body's delicate organs while we are carrying out our daily activities — walking, jumping, running or bumping into things.

Insulation — triglycerides form a layer around the body, which conserves heat to keep the body temperature constant.

The triglycerides also serve as the body's reserve of the valuable essential fatty acids, LA and LNA which are required for the structure and functions of the membranes and the precursors of prostaglandins.

An important function of the triglycerides is to convert excess sugar to fat should this be necessary. The brain needs glucose to function, but sugars in excess are toxic so can be converted to triglycerides that are less harmful in large quantities. So the triglycerides provide a safety net for the body by converting a potentially toxic substance (excess sugar) into a neutral one. It is therefore very easy to become overweight (fat) without actually consuming large amounts of fat.

Excess triglycerides cause problems, and are associated with disease. High TG levels in the blood are associated with heart disease and are produced by overeating and especially by a high intake of refined sugars in the diet. Being overweight correlates to high triglycerides and high cholesterol levels both of which correlate to cardiovascular problems, high blood pressure, heart and kidney failure. High blood triglyceride levels increase the tendency of blood cells to clump together, decreasing the amount of oxygen the blood can carry and increasing the risk of all degenerative disease, including cancer.

'FAT FREE' DIET FOODS

This is probably a good place to mention the 'fat free' and 99% fat free products that have bombarded our supermarket shelves over the last few years. Many people, those trying to lose weight in particular, pay exorbitant prices for these ready made meals, biscuits, cakes and other products in the belief that they won't make them fat because they don't contain fat. These foods may be low in fat, but they are usually high in sugars and as you now know, the body will convert excess sugar, which could be harmful, to fat, which, although may also be harmful, is a safer alternative. It is no wonder then that unsuccessful dieters become depressed and anxious. You should discourage clients from using these products and encourage going back to what nature intended and that is to eat plenty of vegetables, fruit and wholegrains.

SUPPLEMENTS

There are many different vitamin supplements available and the diversity of choice is astounding. Not all vitamins are the same and not all companies are the same so always purchase on recommendation from a nutritionally qualified therapist or from good health food stores. I would not recommend you buy from mail order companies or from supermarkets or decide by price alone. The most expensive is not always the best and the cheapest may be full of fillers and binders and not much of the nutrient you really want. Look at labels carefully. Many capsules are made from gelatin and are unsuitable for vegetarians. Some weight reduction supplements may contain animal derived thyroid, which again would be unsuitable for some people. Many children's supplements contain artificial colours, flavourings and sugar! So take care when buying supplements.

It would be wonderful if we could get all the nutrients we needed for good health from the food offered to us in our stores. Unfortunately, I believe that due to intensive farming that leaves our soil nutrient deficient, and the ever increasing desire for fast and convenient foods, that that is just not possible. Combined with an increased nutrient requirement due to modern living, we all need some basic form of supplementation. There have been many studies carried out recently showing that on average our fruit and vegetables have 60 per cent *less* vitamin and mineral content than they had just 50 years ago.

I feel that no one is exempt from taking supplements these days. The young at school, the pressured businessman, the busy housewife, in pregnancy, during the menopause, the elderly, the competitive sportsman and those recouping from illness, all require to be optimally nourished. The Bateman Report published in 1985 found more than 85 per cent of people who generally thought they ate a well balanced diet failed to meet RDA levels. That report was 16 years ago and there is little sign that the diet of the nation has improved. I rather feel if anything it has declined still further.

Vitamins

What exactly are they?

Vitamins are organic substances obtained from food or dietary supplements.

Main function

To sustain life.

What do vitamins do?

Vitamins are components of our enzyme systems which, acting like the spark plugs in your car, energise and regulate our metabolism, keeping us tuned up and running at high performance. Although taken in minute amounts compared to the macronutrients and micronutrients a deficiency in even one vitamin can endanger the whole human body.

Vitamins need not be digested but liberated from food. Vitamins give us vitality and are needed not only for good health and a strong immune system but also to be used as co-enzymes to allow other chemical reactions to take place in the body. In metabolism for example, we need good supplies of the B vitamins, or our metabolism will be sluggish. Deficiencies in vitamins give us many symptoms and if we have the symptoms long enough they may result in disease. We all know the story about the British sailors who became sick on the long sea crossings at the beginning of the 20th Century because of lack of fresh fruit and vegetables. When given fresh limes they recovered quickly. It was then that vitamin C was discovered. This was in 1936 and since then many more vitamins have been isolated and there are still many more to be discovered.

HOW MUCH TO TAKE?

Figures are always being updated for vitamin and mineral supplements and it is sometimes hard to keep up to date with all the new information. The Department of Health asked the Committee on Medical Aspects of Food Policy (COMA) to set up a panel of experts to look the various figures and give a new set of updated figures. These are collectively known as Dietary Reference Values. So as well as RDA (Recommended Daily Allowances) figures we also have the following guidelines for supplements:

- ◆ EAR   Estimated Average Requirement
- ◆ RNI   Recommended Nutrient Intake
- ◆ LNI   Lowest Nutrient Intake
- ◆ SI   Safe Intake
- ◆ RDA   Recommended Daily Allowance

The publication of these new dietary guidelines reflects the fact that at long last the health authorities have accepted that everyone's need are different and some people need more of one nutrient than others.

In addition to the above there are also SONAs — Suggested Optimal Nutritional Allowances.[41] Dr. Emanuel Cheraskin and colleagues from the University of Alabama worked for fifteen years studying 13,500 people living in six regions of America. Each participant completed an in depth questionnaire and were given physical, dental, eye and other examinations as well as numerous clinical tests for dietary analysis. The object was to find which nutrient intake levels were associated with the highest health ratings. The results consistently revealed that the healthiest individuals, meaning those with the fewest clinical signs and symptoms, were taking supplements and eating a diet rich in nutrients relative to calories. The researchers found that the intake of nutrients associated with optimal health was often ten or more times higher than the RDA levels. On the basis of this evidence the SONAs were developed. These levels are more likely to be the kind of intake you need to maintain optimum health. These are the levels I usually use in my pracatice. Not all vitamins and minerals have SONAs but I have indicated the ones that have for your information, together with the RDAs.

Vitamins can be put into two groups. The water-soluble vitamins of the B complex group and vitamin C and the fat-soluble vitamins A, D, E and K. The main difference between these two groups of vitamins is that the water soluble vitamins need to be ingested every day as the body cannot store them whereas the fat soluble vitamins are stored in the body and need not be ingested every day. The storage of these vitamins is one function of the liver.

THE FAT SOLUBLE VITAMINS
VITAMIN A *(Retinol, Beta-Carotene)*

Main Deficiency symptoms

Poor night vision, dry flaky skin, acne, frequent colds or infections and mouth ulcers.

Main food sources

Fish liver oil, liver, eggs and dairy produce (especially margarine that is usually fortified) carrots, and all yellow fruits and vegetables.

Main functions:

An essential vitamin for reproduction, for the maintenance of the skin and for supporting the immune system.

Liver is an excellent source of vitamin A. However, it should be remembered that the liver is an organ of detoxification not only for us but also for animals. When we eat liver, we are ingesting the stored medications, antibiotics, and hormones that animal may have been given throughout its life. I would suggest that eating animal liver should be restricted to once a fortnight. On the other hand, by eating, carrots, red peppers, aubergines, tomatoes and other fruits and vegetables, we are taking in good amounts of beta-carotene, which the body can synthesise into vitamin A if required. This is a much safer way of getting adequate amounts of vitamin A into the body, as beta-carotene is water soluble and non-toxic.

Vitamin A is an antioxidant and is available to us in two forms. Pre-formed vitamin A known as retinol which is only found in foods of animal origin, and pro-vitamin A, which is obtained from fruits and vegetables as well as animal origin, and also known as carotene.

Vitamin A as Retinol	ADULTS	CHILDREN
RDA	600mcgRE	350–500mcgRE
SONA	2,000mcgRE	800–1,000mcgRE
Therapeutic	2250–6000mcgRE	1250mcgRE
Cautions	3000mcg maximum if pregnant or trying	Toxicity may occur if doses exceed 4000mcgRE daily

VITAMIN D
(Calciferol, Viosterol, Ergosterol, Sunshine vitamin)

Main Deficiency symptoms

Joint pain or stiffness, lack of energy, rheumatism or arthritis, hair loss, rickets in children and osteomalacia in adults.

Main food sources

Fish liver oils, sardines, herring, salmon, tuna, milk, meat and eggs. We also obtain vitamin D from sunlight. Ultraviolet light acts on the oils of the skin to produce the vitamin, which is then absorbed into the body.

Main functions:

Known as the sunshine vitamin, vitamin D is an antioxidant and promotes absorption of calcium and phosphate from food, necessary for strong bones and teeth. It is needed for the correct function of thyroid and parathyroid glands, promoting release of calcium from bones and ensuring proper distribution in body as well as increases uptake of mineral by bone. As a fat-soluble vitamin, we do not need it every day, as it is stored in our liver.

Causes of deficiency are lack of meat, fish and dairy products in the diet, and lack of exposure to sunlight.

It is the most toxic of all the vitamins but also the most stable. Calcium and phosphorus are needed for the utilisation of vitamin D, and vitamins A, C and E, the antioxidants, protect vitamin D.

VITAMIN D	ADULTS	CHILDREN
RDA	10mcg	10mcg
SONA	10–20mcg	10–20mcg
Therapeutic	10–25mcg	5–12mcg
Cautions	1250mcg potentially toxic	

VITAMIN E
(Tocopherol)

Main Deficiency symptoms

Easy bruising, exhaustion after light exercise, slow wound healing, lack of sex drive, varicose veins and loss of muscle tone.

Main food sources

Soya beans, unrefined corn oils, broccoli, Brussel sprouts, green leafy vegetables, sunflower seeds, sesame seeds, peanuts, whole grain cereals, wheat germ, tuna and sardines.

Main functions:

Vitamin E is an antioxidant, which prevents oxidation of fat compounds as well as vitamins A, C and D, selenium, and two sulphur amino acids. It protects the cardiovascular system, prevents thrombosis, arteriosclerosis, thrombophlebitis, increases HDLs, maintains healthy blood vessels, reduces the oxygen needs of muscles, promotes white call resistance to infection, and potentiates the action of selenium. Vitamin E enhances the activity of vitamin A and is important as a vasodilator and an anticoagulant.

Causes of deficiency are fat malabsorption; high intake of refined oils; alcoholism; intestinal surgery; cirrohosis of the liver and coeliac disease. Do not use high doses if taking Warfarin or other anti-coagulant drugs.

Taking vitamin E may initially raise blood pressure as it reduces blood clotting, so gradual increase in dosage recommended with cardiovascular problems.

VITAMIN E	ADULTS	CHILDREN
RDA	3–4mg	0.3mg
SONA	100–1000mg	70mg
Therapeutic	100–1000mg	70–100mg
Cautions	Toxicity – non reported below 2000mg long term use and 35,000mg short term use	

VITAMIN K
(Phylloquinone)

Main Deficiency symptoms:

Excess bleeding (nosebleeds), abnormal blood clotting, fall in prothrombin content of blood.

Main food sources

Cabbage family, lettuce, beans, peas, watercress, potatoes, tomatoes, asparagus and corn oil. Also synthesised by gut flora.

Main functions:

The main function of vitamin K is that of blood clotting, the formation of prothrombin (a blood clotting chemical) and normal liver function. It helps in preventing internal bleeding and haemorrhages and aids in reducing excessive menstrual flow, as well as promoting proper blood clotting.

Causes of deficiency are birth — before sufficient intestinal flora is present to produce vitamin K. Other causes are anticoagulant therapy, liver cirrhosis and viral hepatitis.

Supplementing vitamin K is usually unnecessary, as there is an abundance of natural vitamin K generally in the diet. However, after taking a course of antibiotics, a course of vitamin K could be considered. If taking the Pill or HRT supplementing vitamin K should be avoided as vitamin K is involved in blood clotting and the risk of blood clots is increased by synthetic hormones. There is never any need to restrict dietary forms of vitamin K from cauliflower and other vegetables, but no additional supplements should be taken

VITAMIN K	ADULTS	CHILDREN
RDA	Not established	Not established
SONA	55–80mcg	45mcg
Therapeutic	300mcg (after antibiotics)	45mcg (after antibiotics)
Cautions	The synthetic form of Vitamin K – Menadone – is best avoided	The synthetic form of Vitamin K – Menadone – is best avoided

REMEMBER
Vitamins A, D. E & K – are fat-soluble vitamins that are stored in the liver.
As supplements they need to be taken with meals containing fats and minerals to be properly absorbed.

THE WATER SOLUBLE VITAMINS.
B1 *(Thiamine)*

Main functions:

Essential for energy production, brain function and digestion. Acts as co-enzyme in converting glucose into energy, involved in production of acetylcholine, involved in protein metabolism.

Main food sources

Dried Brewer's yeast, yeast extract, brown rice, wheatgerm, nuts, pork, wheat bran, soya flour, whole grains, especially germinating grains and liver.

Main Deficiency symptoms

Tender muscles, fatigue, stomach pains, burning or numbness in legs/ toes/soles, eye pains, insomnia, confusion, irritability, poor concentration, poor memory, and constipation.

Causes of deficiency

A diet high in refined carbohydrates, pregnancy, breast-feeding, fever, surgery, physical and mental stress, alcohol, overuse of antacid drugs.

Therapeutic uses

Beri-beri (a deficiency disease of the nervous system caused by diet of refined rice), improvement of mental ability, indigestion, improving heart function, alcoholism, lumbago, sciatica, neuralgia, and facial paralysis.

Notes

Cooking, smoking, drinking, stress, and antacid tablets deplete it in the body.
Most beneficial as part of a B Complex formula

B1 *(Thiamine)*	ADULTS	CHILDREN
RDA	0.8–1mg	0.4–1.1mg
SONA	3.5–9.2mg	3.1–3.3mg
Therapeutic	25–100mg	12.5–50mg
Cautions	No known toxicity.	No known toxicity

B2 *(Riboflavin)*

Main functions:

Acts as co-enzymes that are concerned with conversation of fats, sugars and protein into energy; needed to maintain body tissues and mucous membranes; acts in conversion of tryptophan to nicotinic acid, helps to regulate body acidity.

Main food sources

Yeast extract, brewer's yeast, milk, cheese, organ meats (especially liver), wheatgerm, eggs, legumes, mushrooms, watercress, cabbage and asparagus.

Main Deficiency symptoms

Cracks and sores in the corners of mouth and eyes, bloodshot, tired eyes, feeling of grit under eyelids, conjunctivitis, cataracts, photophobia, inflamed tongue and lips, scaling of skin around face, dully oily hair and hair loss, trembling, sluggishness, dizziness, insomnia, slow learning.

Causes of deficiency

The causes of deficiency are alcohol; contraceptive pill; smoking; and faulty dietary habits.

Therapeutic uses

Therapeutic uses are mouth ulcers, gastric and duodenal ulcers, eye ulceration and cataracts, eczema, hypothyroidism, certain cancers, nervous disorders, vaginitis, fevers, stress of injury or surgery, malabsorption.

Notes

Heat, ultraviolet light, the birth control pill and alkaline agents (baking powder) deplete it in the body. Most beneficial as part of a B Complex formula

B2 *(Riboflavin)*	**ADULTS**	**CHILDREN**
RDA	1.1.–1.3mg	0.4–1.1mg
SONA	1.8mg-2.5mg	1.8–2.0mg
Therapeutic	25–100mg	12.5–50mg
Cautions	No known toxicity	No known toxicity

B3 *(Niacin)*

Main functions:

Acts as coenzymes responsible for cell respiration. Produces energy from sugars, fats and proteins. Crucial for brain function (involved with production of serotonin). Component of GTF – helps maintain normal blood sugar levels. Maintains healthy skin, nerves, brain, tongue, digestive system and involved in the synthesis of sex hormones.

Main food sources

Yeast extract, brewer's beast, wheat bran, turkey and chicken, fish, whole grains (especially sprouting grains) peanuts, mushrooms and milk products.

Main Deficiency symptoms

Dementia, depression, anxiety, irritability, digestive disturbances, insomnia, dermatitis, rashes, acne, rough inflamed skin, inflamed mouth, tremors, allergies. Pellagra is major deficiency disease affecting skin, digestive and nervous systems.

Causes of deficiency

Alcohol; anti-leukemia drugs. Pellagra develops in areas where maize (corn) is staple diet.

Therapeutic uses

Schizophrenia; alcoholism, tobacco addiction., acne, arthritis, reducing blood cholesterol, digestive problems, diarrhoea, migraine, and insomnia.

Notes

Very stable but losses occur during cooking and food processing. Destroyed by alcohol. Antibiotics, coffee, tea, the birth control pill deplete it in the body. Most beneficial as part of a B Complex formula and additional chromium (to make GTF). B3 is available in two forms, *Niacin* which may cause flushing and *niacinamine*.

B3	ADULTS	CHILDREN
RDA	13–17mg	5–10gm
SONA	25–30mg	25mg
Therapeutic	50–150mg	25–50mg
Cautions	No known toxicity below 3000mg	

B5 *(Pantothenic Acid)*

Main functions:

Involved in energy production, production of anti-stress hormones, controlling fat metabolism, formation of anti-bodies, maintaining healthy nerves and maintains health of skin and hair.

Main food sources

All animal and plant tissue (named from 'panthos' meaning everywhere), mushrooms, avocados, whole wheat, lentils and eggs.

Main Deficiency symptoms

Burning feet, poor concentration, apathy, fatigue, restlessness, vomiting, asthma, allergies, muscle cramps, loss of appetite and indigestion.

Causes of deficiency

Stress and antibiotics.

Therapeutic uses

Rheumatoid arthritis, allergic reactions, stress, nerve disorders and epilepsy and for detoxifying drugs especially antibiotics.

Notes

Destroyed by heat, food processing extremes of acidity and alkalinity (vinegar and baking powder). Biotin and folic acid aid absorption. Most beneficial as part of a B Complex formula.

B5 *(Pantothenic Acid)*	ADULTS	CHILDREN
RDA	3–7mg	3–7mg
SONA	25mg	10mg
Therapeutic	50–300mg	25–150mg
Cautions	None known below 100 times RDA level	

B6 *(Pyridoxine)*

Main functions:

Acts as coenzymes in protein metabolism. Needed for synthesis of certain brain chemicals and conversion of tryptophan to B3. Crucial to blood formation, energy production and EFA metabolism. Also has anti-depressant and anti-allergy functions.

Main food sources

Brewer's yeast, wheat bran, yeast extract, animal and dairy produce, bananas, broccoli, red kidney beans, watercress, cauliflower and cabbage.

Main Deficiency symptoms

Irritability, depression, bloatedness, fluid retention, hair loss, cracks around mouth, numbness, muscle cramps, slow learning, pregnancy sickness, allergies, tingling hands, poor dream recall and memory, flaky skin.

Causes of deficiency

Contraceptive pill, many drugs (penicillamine), alcohol, smoking, fasting and reducing diets.

Therapeutic uses

PMT, depression, disorders caused by contraceptive pill, morning sickness, travel sickness, radiation sickness, fluid retention, facial dermatitis, anaemia, bronchial asthma, skin allergies, diabetes, kidney stones.

Notes

Works synergistically with zinc. Most beneficial as part of a B Complex formula to balance. Alcohol, smoking birth control pill, processed foods and a high protein diet will all deplete this vitamin in the body. If taken without other B vitamins a tolerance to B6 may be built up and deficiency of other B vitamins arises

B6 *(Pyridoxine)*	ADULTS	CHILDREN
RDA	1.2–1.4 mg	0.5–1mg
SONA	10–25mg	2–5mg
Therapeutic	50–250mg	25–125mg
Cautions	Toxicity reported in doses over 1000mg taken alone.	

B12 *(cyanocobalamin)*

Main functions:

Essential for production of red blood cells which carry oxygen to all other cells in the body protects our nerves, needed for making use of protein, needed for synthesis of DNA, detoxifies tobacco smoke and other toxins in food.

Main food sources

Oysters, pig's liver and kidney, sardines, pork, beef, lamb, white fish, eggs, cheese. Only found in foods of animal origin with the exception of spirulina algae.

Main Deficiency symptoms

Both B12 and folic acid deficiencies have been shown to cause psychiatric illness such as dementia. Smooth sore tongue, nerve degeneration (tremors, numbness, psychosis, mental deterioration), anaemia, lassitude and weakness, menstrual disorders.

Causes of deficiency

Non-absorption due to lack of intrinsic factor in gastric mucosa (and/or HCl) produces pernicious anaemia, intestinal parasites, veganism, pregnancy, ageing, alcohol, and heavy smoking.

Therapeutic uses

Pernicious anaemia (by injection from GP), moodiness, poor memory, paranoia, mental confusion, tiredness, poor appetite.

Notes

There have been no reported problems with B12 supplementation in the oral form although rarely an allergic reaction may arise with an injected dose. B12 is not readily absorbed and as such can be bought in a nugget form, which is placed under the tongue for more efficient absorption.*(Appendix I)*

B12 *(cyanocobalamin)*	ADULTS	CHILDREN
RDA	1.5mcg	0.3–1.2mcg
SONA	2–3mcg	2mcg
Therapeutic	5–100mcg	2.5–25mcg
Cautions	None reported	

FOLIC ACID

Main functions:

Helps regulate histamine levels, critical during pregnancy for child's development, Involved in function of RNA and DNA in protein synthesis and red blood formation.

Main food sources

Chicken livers, bulgar wheat, spinach, red kindly beans, wheatgerm, orange juice, avocado, chickpeas, broccoli, beetroot, raspberries, peanuts asparagus, cashew nuts.

Main Deficiency symptoms

Anaemia (linked with B12), weakness, fatigue, breathlessness, irritability, insomnia, forgetfulness, cracked lips, prematurely greying hair, and depression. In pregnancy, can result in miscarriage, premature birth, toxemia, and possibly spina bifida.

Causes of deficiency

Pregnancy, contraceptive pill, old age, certain drugs. 50–90% lost in cooking.

Therapeutic uses

When planning a pregnancy, pregnancy problems, mental deterioration, psychosis, malabsorption problems.

Notes

There are many studies showing that if women take folic acid before conceiving and in the early days or pregnancy that Neural Tube Defects may be prevented. Works best with B12 and as part of a B Complex formula. High temperature and light, food processing also causes losses of folic acid. Supplementation of folic acid can mask a B12 deficiency anaemia, therefore should not be taken without a basic intake of B12.

FOLIC ACID	ADULTS	CHILDREN
RDA	200mcg	50–150mcg
SONA	400–1000mcg	300mcg
Therapeutic	400–1000mcg	25–300mcg
Cautions	Seldom reported, but in some cases more than 15mg daily can lead to loss of appetite, nausea, flatulence, abdominal distention and sleep disturbances.	

BIOTIN

Main functions:

Coenzyme in many body actions including: metabolism of proteins, fats and carbohydrates, maintaining healthy skin, hair, sweat glands, nerves, and bone marrow.

Main food sources

Found in all animal and plant tissues, especially yeasts, liver and kidney and milk produce, watermelon, cauliflower, sweetcorn, almonds, eggs and tomatoes.
Large quantities are also produced by healthy intestinal bacteria.

Main Deficiency symptoms

Fatigue, depression, nausea, sleepiness, smooth pale tongue, loss of appetite, muscular pains, loss of reflexes, hair loss.
In babies : dermatitis, scaly skin anaemia and diarrhoea.

Causes of deficiency

Stress, antibiotics, feeding new born child with unfortified dried milk, excessive intake of raw egg-whites (avedin, a protein in uncooked egg induces biotin deficiency).

Therapeutic uses

Seborrheic dermatitis, Leiner's disease, alopecia, scalp disease, skin complaints, candidiasis.

Notes

Most beneficial as part of a B Complex formula with magnesium and manganese. Fried food destroys biotin. Biotin is also known as vitamin H, and coenzyme R. All cells contain some biotin, with large quantities in the liver and kidneys.

BIOTIN	ADULTS	CHILDREN
RDA	10–200mcg	10–200mcg
SONA	50–200mcg	50–200mcg
Therapeutic	50–200mcg	25–100mcg
Cautions	None reported	None reported

CHOLINE

Main functions:

Fat stabilising agent – as component of lecithin helps to break down accumulating fats in the liver and facilitates movement of fats into cells, pre-cursor of betaine, needed in metabolism, helps make neurotransmitter acetylcholine, essential for health of myelin sheaths. Protects the lungs.

Main food sources

Present in all living cells. Best sources lecithin granules, desiccated liver, eggs, fish, liver, wheatgerm, brewer's yeast.

Main Deficiency symptoms

No specific symptoms, but lack can lead to fatty liver, nerve degeneration, high blood pressure, atherosclerosis, thrombosis, high blood cholesterol, senile dementia, reduced resistance to infection.

Causes of deficiency

Alcohol, birth control pills.

Therapeutic uses

Cardiovascular problems, alcoholism, diabetes, liver and kidney diseases.

Notes

Alcohol and the birth control pill will deplete body. As choline is synthesised in the body it is not a true vitamin and is therefore known as a semi-essential nutrient. Choline is also known as lipotropic factor. Works well with B5 and lithium.

CHOLINE	ADULTS	CHILDREN
RDA	None	None
SONA	None	None
Therapeutic	25–150mg	12.5–75mg
Cautions	None Known	

VITAMIN C *(Ascorbic Acid)*

Main functions:

Antioxidant – protects other nutrients, prevents cellular damage, detoxifies heavy metals and carcinogens, makes collagen, and keeps skin, bones, joints and arteries healthy. Vital for supporting immune system, antibody production, it is a natural 'anti-histamine', reduces cholesterol levels, aids absorption of iron, produces anti-stress hormones, and activates folic acid.

Main food sources

All fruits and vegetables, especially guava fruit, peppers, cantaloupe melon, pimientos, papaya, strawberries, Brussel sprouts, grapefruit juice and sprouted seeds and beans.

Main Deficiency symptoms

Frequent colds and infections, lack of energy, allergies, bleeding gums, easy bruising, nose bleeds, slow wound healing, anaemia, premature ageing. Deficiency disease *scurvy*.

Causes of deficiency

Diet high in refined foods, low in fruit and vegetables, poor absorption, stress, alcohol, infections, ageing, drugs (aspirin & barbiturates), contraceptive pill, antibiotics.

Therapeutic uses

Iron deficiency anaema, viral infections, exposure to pollutants, wound healing, recovery from surgery/fractures, dental/gum disease, respiratory problems, alcoholism, arthritis, anti-histamine, cancer, gastrointestinal problems.

Notes

Vitamin C is available in various forms. The most popular form of Vitamin C is as ascorbic acid, which is mildly acidic. This can be bought in tablets or in power form. I prefer the latter which can then be added to bottled water and drank throughout the day. In this way you are getting the benefit of the vitamin and the water.

Calcium ascorbic and Magnesium ascorbic are probably more easily tolerated but in amounts excess of 5g could neutralise stomach acid which is necessary for protein breakdown. If you want to take in excess of 5g of this type of Vitamin C, then it should not be taken with food.

Vitamin C also affects oestrogen. 1g turns low dose contraceptive pill into a high dose, so no more than 500mg should be taken.

High doses can lead to loose bowels. This is not a sign of toxicity but a sign of 'bowel tolerance' of which we are all different. Can be used as a natural laxative in this way.

Lead, copper, aluminium, cadmium (other people's cigarette smoke) mercury, smoking, alcohol, drugs, barbecued food, sun-bed use, pesticides and many other pollutants will deplete the body.

VITAMIN C (Ascorbic Acid)	ADULTS	CHILDREN
RDA	40mg	25–35mg
SONA	400–1000mg	150mg
Therapeutic	1000–10000mg	150–1000mg
Cautions	If you wish to take high doses of Vitamin C – then up to 'bowel tolerance' is a good indicator.	

MINERALS and TRACE MINERALS

What exactly are they?

Inorganic substances mined from the earth.

Main function

They perform functions necessary to life, for example regulating metabolic processes and building tissue.

What do minerals do?

Our bodies are made up of two fundamentally different groups of substances; organic and inorganic.

Organic substances are produced by the chemical reactions of life. They are created, broken down, and recreated in our bodies from the constituents of the food we eat, and the air we breathe forming the dazzling array of molecular structures we need in order to live – nerves, skin, organs and muscles.

Organic structures by their very nature exist in a state of flux, participating in a continual series of chemical transformations, with one succeeding another like the generations of a family. Organic structures are proteins, vitamins, carbohydrates and fats and thanks to them we can grow and multiply, adapt and evolve.

On the other hand, there is no known way in which our bodies can create or break down inorganic substances. These unchanging chemicals are called minerals and trace minerals. They existed long before organic life first appeared on Earth and will exist long after it has vanished. Yet the role these substances play in sustaining the dynamic, ever changing processes of life is invaluable. Until recently the way that minerals affected our bodies was very poorly understood and as such they tended to be ignored in favour of other nutrients. It is now clear that without them there would be no life at all.

About 60 different minerals have been identified in the body of which 21 are considered to be 'essential'. Essential minerals, as with essential amino acids and essential fatty acids, are minerals that must be supplied in the food daily, as they cannot be manufactured in the body. Some minerals are required in substantial amounts, often referred to as the gross minerals or the macro-minerals; calcium, magnesium, sodium, potassium and phosphorus. Others are needed in minute or trace amounts but equally important to health which are known as the trace minerals; chromium, iron, manganese, molybdenum, cobalt, copper and zinc. Four minerals tend to be particularly low among western people, calcium, magnesium, zinc and iron.

CALCIUM

Main functions:

Builds and maintains healthy bones and teeth, controls nerve and muscle excitability, controls conduction of nerve impulses, controls muscle contraction, aids blood clotting, controls cholesterol levels, aids B12 absorption, reduces menstrual cramps.

Main food sources

Ricotta cheese, Parmesan cheese, milk, mackerel, salmon and sardines, dried figs, tofu, low fat yogurt, sesame seeds, oats, millet, almonds, kelp, green leafy vegetables, parsley, and pumpkin-seeds.

Main Deficiency symptoms

Rickets (in children), osteomalacia (in adults), bone pain, muscle weakness and cramps, delayed healing of fractures, tetany (twitches and spasms), tooth decay, brittle nails, insomnia or nervousness, joint pain or arthritis, tooth decay, high blood pressure, fragile bones, menstrual cramps, eczema and rheumatoid arthritis.

Causes of deficiency

Low dietary intake, lack of vitamin D, high intake of wheat bran, phosphates, animal fats, oxalic acid, contraceptive pill, corticosteroid drugs, malabsorption due to low stomach acid, coeliac disease, lactose intolerance, diuretic drugs, pregnancy, breast feeding, oestrogen loss after menopause.

Therapeutic uses

Rickets, osteomalacia, osteoporosis, tetany, coeliac disease, allergy complains, detoxify heavy metals, depression, anxiety, panic attacks, insomnia, arthritis, muscle and joint pains, pregnancy, breast feeding.

Notes

Calcium is the most abundant mineral in the body and 99% of this is in the bones and teeth. The remaining 1% is found in the blood and is needed for balanced nerve function, blood clotting, the heart muscles and for enzyme reactions.

Many people think of bone as a hard substance that stops growing when we reach adulthood, and are therefore surprised when they discover that the whole skeleton is in a constant state of flux. The calcium phosphate that gives the bone its hardness is continually forming, dissolving and being reformed. New calcium phosphate deposits are usually built into the protein matrix along the bone shaft while older material is flushed away in the blood to be used for other purposes or excreted by the kidneys in the urine. This constant bone refurbishment allows for growth in the young and ensures that adult bones remain strong and resilient. In this way, an average of 700mg of calcium moves into and out of the bones every day.

The distinction must be made clear regarding weight bearing exercise. Swimming, whilst a fantastic overall exercise, is not a weight bearing exercise as the water is offering protection to the bones. Cycling, another excellent aerobic exercise is again not weight bearing. Weight bearing exercises include walking, jogging, running, climbing stairs and skipping rope.

A number of factors may prevent sufficient calcium from reaching your nerve cells. Excess dietary fibre is one, as it bonds with calcium in the small intestine and prevents it from being absorbed as well as it might. Phytic acid – a substance found in grains – as well as too much fat in your diet have the same effect. Alcohol too prevents your body from utilising calcium by causing the kidney to excrete it in the urine. The result will be too few calcium ions in the nerve cells, which then become over-susceptible to stimuli. In time this could cause the person to become tense, irritable, bad-tempered and highly sensitive 'jumpy' people.

CALCUIM	ADULTS	CHILDREN
RDA	800mg	600mg
SONA	800–1200mg	600–800mg
Therapeutic	800–1200mg	600–800mg
Cautions	None reported from calcium itself but may arise from other factors. Excess Vitamin D in amounts over 25,000ius daily.	

MAGNESIUM — *(Mn)*

Main functions:

Strengthens bones and teeth, promotes healthy muscles so helping them to relax, beneficial for PMS, heart muscles and nervous system. Involved as co-enzymes for many functions in the body and essential for energy production.

Main food sources

Wheatgerm, almonds and cashew nuts, soybeans, whole grains, green leafy vegetables and sesame seeds, potato skins and crab meat.

Main Deficiency symptoms

Depression, muscle tremors or spasms, muscle weakness, insomnia or nervousness, high blood pressure, irregular heart beat, constipation, fits or convulsions, hyperactivity, poor memory, irritability, calcium deposits in soft tissue, e.g. kidney stones.

Causes of deficiency

Low dietary intake due to eating refined foods whose magnesium has been lost in the refining process, and a lack of green leafy vegetables.

Therapeutic uses

Depression, cardiovascular disease, PMS, muscle twitches and spasams.

Notes

Large amounts of calcium in milk products, proteins, fats, oxalates (spinach, rhubarb), phytate (wheat bran and bread) all deplete magnesium from the body. Works well with B1 and B6. Usually taken in conjunction with calcium giving a good balance. There are many forms of magnesium in supplements but the best absorbed is Magnesium Citrate. Works well combined with calcium as a 3:2 calcium:magnesium ratio.

MAGNESIUM	ADULTS	CHILDREN
RDA	300mg	170mg
SONA	375–500mg	200–375mg
Therapeutic	400–800mg	400–800mg
Cautions	None below 1000mg	

SODIUM – *(Na)*

Main functions:

Maintaining intra and extra-cellular water balance, in nerve impulse transmission (with potassium), in all muscle contraction, especially heart muscle, involved in control of acid/alkaline balance in body, active transport of amino acids and glucose into cells.

Main food sources

Table salt, sea salt, yeast extract, bacon, smoked fish, salami, sauces, cornflakes, processed cheese and cheese spread, olives, pickles, many meats, especially the smoked variety, and ready-made meals most other refined and processed foods. *(which should be kept to a minimum)*

Main Deficiency symptoms

Low blood pressure, rapid pulse, dry mouth, mental apathy, loss of appetite, muscle cramps and twitches, dehydration, giving 'sunken' features and sagging skin.

Causes of deficiency

Dehydration due to high temperatures, hard exercise or work, water intoxication – after heavy sweating when thirst is quenched with water containing no sodium. Low blood sodium causes: kidney and liver disease, hormone imbalance, lung cancer or lung infections, meningitis, myxoedema, toxaemia of pregnancy, hyperglycaemia.

In babies — diarrhoea.

Therapeutic uses

Salt replacement corrects the above conditions.

Notes

Your body contains approximately 100 grammes of sodium in the body, a third of which is packed into the bone. A small fraction of the remainder combines with other minerals in the blood to prevent it from clogging. The rest is found in the fluid surrounding the cells, helping to regulate the passage of nutrients, transmissions of nerve impulses, muscle tone and fluid volume. Whilst sodium is a very important mineral, the majority of people consume too much of it. Salt is in abundance in prepared and processed foods and many people also add salt to their cooking and to prepared food. Clients need to be reminded of this and encouraged to cut back of salt intake. Potassium supplements also help to restore the balance as do saunas and regular exercise.

Over-consumption leads to fluid retention, loss of potassium, high blood pressure, stomach ulcers, arteriosclerosis, oedema, weight gain, renal failure, and bronchial asthma.

IS SALT THE SAME AS SODIUM?

Confusingly, nutrition panels on food labels give only sodium content. Salt is actually sodium chloride. Sodium, as a mineral, is essential for a variety of body functions but eating too much, and especially in combination with a low potassium intake, and being overweight, can lead to high blood pressure in older people. High blood pressure increases the risk of stokes and heart disease hence the importance to cut down on salt.

Some foods claim to be 'reduced salt' or 'low salt', but this is pretty meaningless when the nutrition panel only lists the sodium content. As a consumer, you might think this is a plot to keep you ignorant of the true amount of salt you are eating. Amazingly enough it is actually illegal to give the amount of salt in a particular food on the nutrition panel!.

Whatever the motives of the government and the food industry, you can work out how much salt is in your food by a simple sum.

How much salt in your food?
To calculate the salt content in the food you purchase multiply the 'sodium' content by 2.5

Or you can memorise the daily maximum amount of sodium or salt recommended in the example below.

| How much salt and sodium should you eat? ||
Daily Salt	Daily Sodium
Men – less than 7g per day Women – less than 5g per day	Men – less than 2.5g per day Women – less than 2g per day

Deficiency is rare, problems arising from the body's tendency to retain sodium leading to high blood pressure, heart disease, oedema and kidney disease.

SALT SUBSTITUTES

Most salt substitutes mix ordinary sale (i.e. sodium chloride) with potassium chloride and/or magnesium sulphate (and other ingredients, such as anti-caking agents), so do not be fooled into thinking you are avoiding salt altogether. Products vary widely in the amount of sodium they contain. Reduced sodium 'salts' can contain 50% salt, but very low sodium products may contain only 0.9g per 100g sodium, compared with 38.9g in ordinary salt. Some people detect an aftertaste with potassium products in particular.

THE SODIUM/POTASSIUM RATIO

Food processing removes the potassium found naturally in foods. Our bodies need potassium to keep sodium in balance. The best sources of potassium are vegetables, fruit fish and lean meat. These fresh foods also leave less room for salty, processed foods in your diet. As much as 80% of our salt intake can come from processed and 'ready made' foods.

HOW MUCH SALT IS IN COMMON FOODS?

High Salt foods	Moderate to Low Salt Foods
Table/cooking salt	Fresh fruit and vegetables
Cured/smoked meat	Eggs
Smoked fish	Meat
Canned meat	Game
Cottage cheese	Poultry
Salted butter/margarine/spreads	Fresh fish
Savoury crackers/crisps	Milk
Salted nuts/savoury snacks	Oatmeal and oats
Some sweet biscuits	Pulses
Baked beans	Dried fruit
Canned vegetables	Nuts
Olives	Unsalted butter and low-salt
Sauces	spreads
(ketchup, Worcestershire,	Breakfast cereals without added
brown, and soya sauce)	salt
	(puffed wheat, Shredded Wheat,
	porridge oats)
	Brown rice
	Wholemeal flour and pasta

RECOMMENDATIONS FOR CONTROLLING SALT INTAKE.

♦ Replace canned, pre-packaged, convenience, take-away and ready-made meals with freshly cooked meals made from fresh/frozen vegetables, fish poultry and meat.

♦ Eat more fruit, vegetable and low-salt starchy foods such as rice, pasta, potatoes and bread as part of a balanced diet.

♦ Gradually cut down on the salt you add during cooking and at the table.

Taste buds respond rapidly to salt – the more you have, the more you want. Gradually cutting down results in what you once found tasty becoming unpleasantly salty. It sounds simple, and it is – if you cut down very gradually you won't even notice it. Think of the health benefits.

POTASSIUM

Main functions:

Essential for healthy nerves and muscles, maintains fluid balance in the body, relaxes muscles, helps secretion of insulin for blood sugar control, enables nutrients and waste products to enter and leave cells, maintains heart functioning and stimulates peristalsis to encourage proper movement of food through the digestive tract.

Main food sources

Kelp, Brewer's yeast, raisins, peanuts, dates, vegetables and fruits, wheatgerm, bananas, avocado, dandelion coffee, prunes, grapes, whole grains and nuts, blackstrap molassas, baked potatoes, cantaloupe melon, dried peaches and prunes, tomato juice, low fat yogurt, salmon, apricots, herring.

Main Deficiency symptoms

Muscle weakness and loss of muscle tone, fatigue, constipation, mental apathy, poor reflexes, nervous disorders, arthritis, and irregular heartbeat, and low blood sugar.

Causes of deficiency

An excess of sodium may lead to an increased intake of potassium to maintain the correct water balance in the body. Potassium is easily absorbed and excreted, unless there is some kidney malfunction. Therefore dietary excess is not usually a problem. However, diets high in fat, refined sugars and over-salted foods may lead quickly to a state of potassium deficiency. As we age our potassium levels drop substantially and this is one of the main reasons for the weakness and decline in strength of the elderly.

Therapeutic uses

Muscle weakness, pins and needles, irritability, nausea, vomiting, diarrhoea, swollen abdomen, cellulite, confusion, mental apathy.

Notes

Magnesium helps to hold potassium in cells.

POTASSIUM	ADULTS	CHILDREN
RDA	2000mg	1600mg
SONA	2000mg	1600mg
Therapeutic	200–3500mg	200–1600mg
Cautions	Over 18,000mg Cardiac arrest may occur	

MANGANESE – *(Mn)*

Main functions:

Cofactor in over 20 enzyme systems involving growth, health of nervous system, energy production and health of joints, female sex hormones, production of thyroxin, cofactor for vitamins B, C and E, maintenance of healthy bones, stimulates glycogen storage in liver.

Main food sources

Seeds, nuts and grains, green leafy vegetables, beetroot, pineapple, bran, wheat, egg yolk, kelp, nuts, tropical fruit and black tea.

Main Deficiency symptoms

Muscle twitches, childhood 'growing pains', dizziness or poor sense of balance, fits or convulsions, sore knees and joints.

Causes of deficiency

High intakes of refined/processed foods, long-term zinc deficiency, rarely due to excess copper intake, alcohol, malabsorption, and certain antibiotics.

Therapeutic uses

Schizophrenia, anaemia, zinc and other deficiency conditions, blood sugar problems, cartilage problems, allergies and fatigue.

Notes

Like a number of vitamins and minerals complete deficiency of manganese is virtually impossible, because of its presence in so many foods. However, there are widespread deficiencies in the western world. Depleted by antibiotics, alcohol, refined foods and excesses of calcium and phosphorus. Manganese citrate a good source.

MANGANESE	ADULTS	CHILDREN
RDA	3.5mg	2.5mg
SONA	5mg	2.5mg
Therapeutic	2.5–15mg	2.5–5mg
Cautions	None reported	None reported

CHROMIUM

Main functions:

Forms part of Glucose Tolerance Factor (GTF) to balance blood sugar, helps to normalise hunger and reduce cravings. Essential for heart function and protects DNA and RNA.

Main food sources

Brewers yeast, whole grains especially rye, oysters, green peppers, eggs, liver, beef, mushrooms and molasses.

Main Deficiency symptoms

Excessive or cold sweats, dizziness or irritability after 6 hours without food, need for frequent meals, cold hands, need for excessive sleep or drowsiness during the day, excessive thirst and addicted to sweet foods, arteriosclerosis, improper glucose metabolism, hypoglycemia, diabetes, heart disease, decreased growth, and improper fat metabolism.

Causes of deficiency

High intakes of refined/processed foods.

Therapeutic uses

Imbalances in blood sugar levels, heart disease.

Notes

Widespread deficiencies of chromium have been reported in developed countries. It is believed to be partly due to the use of refined sugar and wheat products, which have between 50 per cent and 94 percent of their chromium removed. Exercise will improve chromium status. Works well with B3 and best bought as a Chromium + B3 together to enhance each other.

CHROMIUM	ADULTS	CHILDREN
RDA	None established	None established
SONA	100mcg	35–50mcg
Therapeutic	20–200mcg	35–50mcg
Cautions	None reported	None reported

COPPER

Main functions:

It is essential for life in small amounts 2g daily is all that is required. It is involved in many enzyme systems including one which protects us from free radicals and is needed to help iron carry out its functions of oxygen transfer to the cells. It helps manufacture a thyroid-stimulating hormone, assists protein manufacture, helps iron to form red cells and assists in the formation of the pigment melanin. Copper helps relieve rheumatism and assists in the metabolism of cholesterol. It is also used for the formation of insulating the myelin sheath around the nerves.

Main food sources

Shellfish especially oysters, organ meats, cereals, dried fruit, almonds, beans and green leafy vegetables. We also take it in by absorbing excess cooper from water pipes, water softeners, fungicides, metal utensils, oestrogen-containing birth control pills and HRT may also elevate blood cooper levels.

Main Deficiency symptoms

General weakness, anaemia, osteoporosis, arthritis, atherosclerosis, heart damage, skin sores, hair loss, digestive problems and diarrhoea.

Causes of deficiency

High doses of zinc may induce copper deficiency.
Excess more likely to be a problem. **Excess symptoms:** hardening of the arteries, high blood pressure, kidney disease, psychosis, early senility and other signs of early aging. Said to be linked to postnatal depression.

Therapeutic uses

Rheumatoid Arthritis

Notes

Copper deficiency is somewhat uncommon because of its abundant availability in our drinking water via copper pipes. In large amounts it is considered toxic. Cooper and zinc are strongly antagonistic so a deficiency in zinc can increase the absorption of copper, as can an over-acidic diet. An excess of copper causes zinc loss.

COPPER	ADULTS	CHILDREN
RDA	None established	None established
SONA	None established	None established
Therapeutic	Unnecessary	Unnecessary
Cautions		

IRON – *(Fe)*

Main functions:

There are between 3 and 4 grams of iron in the body, and more than half of this is used in the blood as a substance called haemoglobin. Transports oxygen and carbon dioxide to and from cells. Component of enzymes, vital for energy production.

Main food sources

Meats, fish, pumpkin seeds, parsley, almonds, brazil and cashew nuts, dates and prunes.

Main Deficiency symptoms

Anaemia, poor vision, insomnia, pale skin, score tongue, fatigue or listlessness, loss of appetite or nausea, heavy periods or blood loss, breathlessness, difficulty is swallowing, general itching, nail deformities, cramping, depression, palpitations and under active thyroid.

Causes of deficiency

Low dietary intake, heavy bleeding, menorrhagia and malabsorption due to lack of stomach acid.

Therapeutic uses

Iron-deficient anaemia generalised itching, impaired mental performance in young, insomnia.

Notes

This chemical is manufactured in the bone marrow and is responsible in turn for the formation of red blood cells. The other half is employed in forming enzymes called cytochromes, which enable the cells to use oxygen in their metabolic pathways. Iron therefore helps the body make full use of its oxygen, both transporting it to where it is needed and then ensuring that it is utilised properly. Every organ in the body is dependent upon oxygen. Therefore if we are iron deficient then every organ in the body will suffer. Amino Acid chelated iron is three times more absorbable than iron sulphate or oxide. Some companies offer a 'gentle' iron that is non-constipating. (*see Appendix I*)

IRON	ADULTS	CHILDREN
RDA	10–14mg	7–10mg
SONA	15mg	7–10mg
Therapeutic	15–25mg	7–10mg
Cautions	None below 1000mg	None below 1000mg

SELENIUM (Se)

Main functions:

Protects the body against toxic metabolites and cancer as anti-oxidant and cofactor of glutathione peroxidase, protects against toxic minerals, maintenance of normal liver function, production of prostaglandins, in male reproduction, maintains health of eyes, hair and skin, anti-inflammatory agent, maintains health of heart, potentiates action of vitamin E and helps produce coenzyme Q.

Main food sources

Organ meats, fish and shellfish, muscle meats, wholegrains, cereals, dairy produce, fruit and vegetables, brazil nuts, puffed wheat, sunflower seeds, brewers yeast, and garlic.

Main Deficiency symptoms

No specific symptoms yet established but seems to be related to liver disease, cancer, cataracts, hart disease, ageing, growth and fertility problems.

Causes of deficiency

High intake of refined/processed foods.
High intake of foods grown on selenium deficient soil.

Therapeutic uses

Arthritis, high blood pressure, angina, hair, nail and skin problems, detoxification of cadmium, arsenic and mercury, cataracts, nutritional muscular dystrophy, liver disease, male infertility, cancer.

Notes

Since the discovery that cancer rates are low in areas with selenium-rich soil, scientists have focused their attention on this trace mineral. As an anti-oxidant, works well with vitamins A, C and E.

SELENIUM	ADULTS	CHILDREN
RDA	70mcg	30mcg
SONA	100mcg	50mcg
Therapeutic	25–100mcg	30–50mcg
Cautions	None below 750mcg	

ZINC *(Zn)*

Main functions:

Essential for bone growth, sexual development, energy production, maintenance of blood sugar levels (as it is needed for insulin production). It is needed to use B6 and vitamin A efficiently, and carries carbon dioxide from the cells to lungs. It maintains acid-alkaline balance in the body and is essential component of prostate, ovaries and testes

Main food sources

Oysters, beef, lamb, sardines, crabmeat, calf's liver, dark turkey meat, brazil nuts, egg yolk, yeast and pumpkin seeds.

Main Deficiency symptoms

Poor sense of taste or smell, white marks on more than two finger nails, frequent infections, stretch marks, acne or greasy skin, low fertility, pale skin, tendency to depression and poor appetite.

Causes of deficiency

Kidney disease, alcoholism, oestrogen also affects zinc levels, the contraceptive pill causes a drop in zinc, as does the high level of natural oestrogen in the body before a period, frequent sexual intercourse in men, high intake of refined/processed foods.

Therapeutic uses

Frequent infections, stretch marks, acne or greasy skin, poor appetite, tendency to depression, low fertility, loss of menstruation.

Notes

Many zinc supplements are on the market. I prefer zinc citrate, or an amino acid chelate. Zinc can also be obtained in liquid form whereby a few drops are added to bottled water and taken throughout the day. Phytates (wheat) and oxalates (rhubarb and spinach) prevent zinc being absorbed. Care must be taken as zinc and copper are highly antagonistic – a high intake of zinc may induce a copper deficiency.

ZINC	ADULTS	CHILDREN
RDA	15mg	7mg
SONA	15–20mg	7mg
Therapeutic	15–50mg	5–10mg
Cautions	Toxicity – 2g or more can cause problems, vomiting and stomach irritation.	

PHOSPHORUS

Main functions:

Forms and maintains bone and teeth, needed for milk secretion, builds muscle tissue and is a component of DNA and RNA, helps maintain pH of the body and aids metabolism and energy production.

Main food sources

Carbonated soft and 'diet' drinks, red meat, and junk food is loaded with phosphorus, additives, Brewers' yeast, wheat bran, Cheddar cheese, brown rice, nuts and eggs.

Main Deficiency symptoms

Calcification causing 'spurs' and imbalance such as osteoporosis, loss of muscle control and strength, trembling, convulsion, high blood pressure, arteriosclerosis and heart disease.

Causes of deficiency

Unlikely to be deficient in phosphorus.

Therapeutic uses

For correct balance of calcium:magnesium:phosphorous

Notes

Phosphorus plays a crucial role in determining how well calcium is absorbed, extracted and distributed in the body. 80% of all the phosphorus in the body is contained in the bones and whenever we speak of calcium's role in bone manufacture we should always include phosphorus in the same breath. This is because the two are stored together in the bone as a compound called calcium phosphate.

PHOSPHORUS	ADULTS	CHILDREN
RDA	800mg	800mg
SONA	None established	None established
Therapeutic	Not usually necessary	Not usually necessary
Cautions	None established	

SULPHUR

Main functions:

Joint protection and repair, antioxidant/free radical scavenger, protection and strengthening of skin, hair and nail tissue, detoxification, heavy metal removal and general connective tissue repair. Helps maintain oxygen balance necessary for proper brain function.

Main food sources

Eggs, onions, garlic, seafood, milk, cabbage, lean beef, dried beans.

Main Deficiency symptoms

Joint aches and pains, frequent infections, poor nails, hair and skin, back pain.

Causes of deficiency

Insufficient intake in the diet, stress, excessive exercise.

Therapeutic uses

Rheumatoid arthritis, after strain or injury, back pain, joint pain, reducing inflammation caused by damage or overuse, improves circulation.

Notes

MSM (*methyl sulfonyl methane*) is a major source of organic sulphur. Preliminary research suggests that MSM may provide significant relief form arthritis and other types of joint injury. Sulphur acts as a very powerful antioxidant. Heavy metals such as lead, mercury and cadmium are very destructive to the body in many ways. Sulphur-containing compounds generally are very effective chelators of heavy metals by latching on to them and assisting their removal from the body. Works well with B-complex group of vitamins and forms part of the tissue building amino acids known as the sulphur containing amino acids.

SULPHUR	ADULTS	CHILDREN
RDA	None reported	None reported
SONA	None	None
Therapeutic	Sufficient protein in diet	Sufficient protein in diet
Cautions	No known toxicity	

ANTI-OXIDANTS

Main functions:

To protect body cells against free radical damage, collagen binding and stabilising, anti-inflammatory, anti-allergic, enhances vitamin C, protects capillaries. Anti-oxidants are substances that can protect another substances from oxidation. Added to foods to keep oxygen from changing that food's colour. Antioxidants include the vitamins A, C, E and the mineral selenium. There are also substances referred to as OPCs which are superantioxidants. These are Pine Bark Extract and Grapeseed Extract, which are even more potent than the anti-oxidants.

Main food sources

Fresh fruits and vegetables preferably organic.

Main Deficiency symptoms

Signs of premature ageing, cataracts, high blood pressure, frequent infections, easy bruising, slow wound healing, varicose veins, loss of muscle tone, infertility.

Causes of deficiency

Lack of dietary intake, stress, smoking, alcohol., coffee, tea, other stimulants.

Therapeutic uses

Protection against heart disease, prevention and treatment of vascular disorders such as varicose veins, phlebitis and haemorrhoids, improved circulation, prevention and treatment of arthritis, preventing allergic reactions such as hay fever and food allergies, protecting the skin from wrinkles and lack of elasticity, promotes healing, protection against eye disorders like cataracts, macular degeneration, diabetic retinopathy, and prevention and treatment of oedema.

Notes

FREE RADICALS

Antioxidants protect the body against free radical damage, but what exactly are free radicals? Free radicals are described as any molecule that has an unpaired electron in its outer sheath. Each of the molecules in our bodies has electrons spinning around them in pairs. These paired electrons keep the molecules in balance. If, for any reason, a molecule loses or gains one of these electrons, it becomes out of balance. Free radicals are these molecules which have become unstable due to their having an unpaired electron.

Cells are made up of many complex molecules and have very specific functions. Free radicals damage cell tissue by stealing electrons from balanced molecules in the cell. They do this in an attempt to bring themselves back into balance. When a molecule loses an electron, it weakens the host cell severely. With excess free radical activity in our bodies, we are destroying more cells than we can create. With cell death we have tissue death which becomes organ death with eventual body death. It all begins with free radicals. Excess free radicals are the direct result of the chemical, emotional, physical and infectious stresses we encounter. Poor diet, smoking, alcohol, exercise, pesticides, emotional upset, and infections all produce free radicals.

There are many types of free radicals. One type results from the cellular energy production system in our body. During normal aerobic cellular metabolism, oxygen and food nutrients are utilised to create ATP, the basic energy molecule. Some free radicals are formed as by-products of this process. These particular free radicals are oxygen molecules with unpaired electrons and are called superoxides. Under normal conditions, these free radicals are kept in check by the antioxidant enzyme, superoxide dismutase. When exposed to stress, the production of these superoxides increases. Excess superoxides are extremely dangerous to cell integrity and work to not only break up cell walls, but also to react with other molecules to form even more toxic free radicals.

To fight free radical damage in our bodies, we need antioxidants, which protect cells against free radical attack. In addition to the well-known antioxidants, Vitamins A, C E and the mineral selenium, we also have superantioxidants.

OPC's (*Oligomeric Proanthocyanidins*) are very powerful antioxidant free radical scavengers. They are as much as 50 times more potent than Vitamin E and 20 times more than Vitamin C. Common supplemental sources of OPCs are Pycnogenol (a patented form of pine bark extract) more commonly known as Pine Bark Extract and Grape Seed Extract.

In addition to their very effective antioxidant effect, Pinebark extract and Grapeseed extract (*Oligomeric Proanthocyanidins*) may also reduce allergic reactions, in part, by inhibiting histamine, the compound most associated with allergic reactions. The ability of OPCs to strengthen collagen may reduce the susceptibility of tissues to allergic processes.

Whilst pine bark and grape seed extracts are excellent sources of OPCs, it is important to understand that OPCs are not the only beneficial compounds found in these two products. On examination of the chemical composition of these two products it is clear that they both contain OPCs, however, the quantity and quality of the OPCs differ. What is also evident is that there are compounds, such as organic acids and catechins in pine bark and gallates in grape seed, that further differentiate these two important materials. Therefore grapeseed extract is not better than pine bark extract and vice versa. Both supplements are important and may be taken together in a complementary way. When looking at the differences between these two products it is like comparing oranges to carrots. Both have similar properties, but both very different and supportive in different ways.

PINE BARK EXTRACT	ADULTS	CHILDREN
RDA	None established	None established
SONA	None established	None established
Therapeutic	30mg	15mg
Cautions	None reported	

GRAPESEED EXTRACT	ADULTS	CHILDREN
RDA	None established	None established
SONA	None established	None established
Therapeutic	100mg	50mg
Cautions	None reported	

CO-ENZYME-Q

Main functions:

To improve the cell's ability to use oxygen.

Main food sources

Fish, meat, peanuts, sesame seeds, walnuts, green beans, spinach, broccoli, soya oil.

Main Deficiency symptoms

Low levels can result in high blood pressure, heart attack, angina, immune system depression, periodontal disease, lack of energy and obesity.

Causes of deficiency

Age, lack of exercise.

Therapeutic uses

Cardiovascular health, hypertension, angina, cardiomyopathy, heart arrhythmia, fatigue, weight control, gum disease, immune function, sports nutrition and antioxidant protection.

Notes

Co-enzyme Q 10 more commonly known as Co-Q-10, is a component of every living cell, and as body levels of Co-Q 10 drop, so does the general status of health. High doses may reduce the effectiveness of the drug warfarin. If taking warfarin, do not take Co-Q-10 without the advice of a physician and also consult the physician if Co-Q-10 is being used prior to starting warfarin therapy.

CO-ENZYME-Q	ADULTS	CHILDREN
RDA	None established	None established
SONA	None established	None establised
Therapeutic	10–90mg per day	
Cautions	Non known	

PHYTOESTROGENS

Many common plant-based foods and herbs contain powerful substances known as phytoestrogens. There are hundreds of active compounds, which largely fall into the following main two categories:- isoflavones and lignans.

What exactly are phytoestrogens?

They are substances found in food that play a protective role in the body.

Main functions

They bind excess oestrogens to a protein made in the blood. These excess oestrogens are either made in the body or taken in from the environment by way of the air we breath, the water we drink and in pesticides, plastics and the contraceptive pill.

What do phytoestrogens actually do?

In order for oestrogen to effect the body, it must enter the cells by binding to certain receptors. Phytoestrogens have the ability to attach to oestrogen's receptor sites. By binding to these receptors, phytoestrogens can block some of the oestrogen circulating in the body from getting into cells. As phytoestrogens are described as 'weak oestrogens' the result is much less oestrogen in the body cells. This may actually help prevent hormonally linked cancers like breast cancer.

GENISTEIN

What exactly is genistein?

Genistein is the best studied of all the isoflavones – a category of phytoestrogens.

3 Main functions

Oestrogen regulating
Cardiovascular benefits
Cell protection.

What does genistein actually do?

Oestrogen regulating

Genistein is a phytoestrogen (a weak oestrogen) and together with another phytoestrogen daizen (also a weak oestrogen) are found in soybeans. Genistein can also be described as an adaptogen. It has the remarkable ability to adapt to the body's needs. Phytoestrogens latch on to the same receptor sites as oestrogen in your body. As the receptor sites become filled with phytoestrogens, which typically have $1/1000^{th}$ or less strength than that of human oestrogen, the resulting blocking would lower the total oestrogenic effect on the body. The excess circulating oestrogen would then be excreted by the body with the fibre that is taken in the diet daily. So whether you are oestrogen dominant or oestrogen deficient, genistein, being an adaptogen, may be of benefit to you. This would include anyone suffering from PMS and menopause symptoms.

Cardiovascular disease

Genistein and diadzein may help prevent cardiovascular disease in various ways, such as preventing free radical oxidation of cholesterol, reducing platelet aggregation, reducing plaque formation, reducing adherence of plaque to artery walls and lowering cholesterol levels.

Cell Protection

Soy isoflavones such as genistein appear to possess many mechanisms that may inhibit cell damage. It may inhibit an enzyme, which stimulates growth of damaged cells, and it may aid in reverting certain damaged cells back into normal cells. Genistein has antioxidant activity and may also inhibit oestrogen-dependent cell damage through blocking excessive oestrogenic activity.

FLAXSEED FIBRE

What exactly is Flaxseed Fibre?

Flaxseed is the best studied of all the ligans – a category of phytoestrogens and it is a fibre.

Main Functions

Reduces heart disease, blood pressure and reduces inflammation of bodily tissues

Prevents constipation and reduces cholesterol levels.

Maintains healthy bones and prevents against cancer and regulates blood sugar.

What does Flaxseed Fibre actually do?

Heart Disease/Blood Pressure/Inflammation

Due to its high level of omega-3 fatty acids, flaxseed is extremely useful in reducing coronary heart disease, blood pressure and inflammation of bodily tissues (see omega-3 fatty acids).

Constipation/Cholesterol levels.

There are two types of fibre available to us in food. Insoluble, which reduces bowel transit time, is good for constipation, and allows fecal matter to be expelled from the body more rapidly and soluble fibre which helps regulate blood glucose and reduces cholesterol levels. Flaxseed is two-thirds insoluble fibre and one-third soluble fibre, so it carries both benefits.

Healthy bones and prevents against cancer

Flaxseed can balance the hormone oestrogen in the body due to its phytoestrogen effects. By taking up the oestrogen receptor sites, the excess oestrogens are carried out of the body. It is now widely accepted by nutritionists that people who consume a fibre rich diet have a lower incidence of hormone-related cancers like breast, endometrial and prostate cancer.

Regulates blood sugar

Fibre regulates our blood sugar by slowing our body's absorption of carbohydrates.

Flaxseed and Linseed are two name for the same oil.

CONVERSION TABLES

1 gram (g) = 1000 milligrams (mg) = 1,000,000 micrograms (mcg)
Most vitamins are measured in milligrams or micrograms.

The fat-soluble vitamins A, D and E are usually measured in International Units (ius) a measurement designed to standardise the various forms of these vitamins that have different potencies.

HERBAL REMEDIES

What exactly are herbs?

Herbs are plants of which the stem is not woody or persistent and which dies down to ground after flowering.

Main functions

The main functions of herbs are for food, medicine, scent, and flavour.

What do herbs do?

Herbs have been used for many thousands of years and are used in many ways for many uses. They are one of the oldest forms of therapy practiced by humans. They can be used as preventative preparations like Echinacea to support the immune system, they can be used as diuretics like Agrimony, or they can be used to support systems of the body, like Black Cohosh and Vixex that support the endocrine system and Rhodiola that supports the nervous system.

They are also used to aid recovery of many everyday ailments — burns, insect bites, scalds, catarrh, diarrhoea and indigestion to mention but a few.

They can be used as suppositories (bolus), which help either draw out toxic poisons or as a carrier for healing agents. They can be taken as capsules, extracts, tinctures or applied externally as creams, compresses, ointments or oils. They can be used in conjunction with hydrotherapy or taken into the body by infusions or syrups for treating coughs, mucus congestion, and sore throats.

We add herbs to our foods for flavour but herbs also have a significant role to play in digestive health, working in several ways on symptoms of digestive disorders. Several herbs in particular play vital roles in good digestion.

Sage contains beneficial properties for the liver and kidneys. Sage has anti-putrefactive and anti-scorbutic properties, especially when cooking meat dishes. It is also said to prevent tooth decay.

It is necessary to add herbs whilst foods are cooking to extract the full potential of their essential oil properties. When meat is cooked it produces a poison called cadaverine. When sage is added, whilst cooking, it prevents the putrefaction of the meat and combats the cadeverine. Our liver will produce anti-toxins to prevent us from being poisoned, but if we continually put pressure on our liver by what we eat, we will eventually have problems with this organ. If you enjoy meat, then adding sage to any dish will support your liver.

Thyme has beneficial properties for easing of stomach cramp. Thyme has antispasmodic properties, especially of the stomach.

The laxative herbs, senna, cascara and tamarind speed up the bowel. However they should only be used for short period since the bowels may become unable to work independently.

Peppermint is a herb that relaxes the gut — helpful for dealing with colic, bloating or wind.

Chamomile and ginger are said to improve the motility of food through the intestinal tract and help reduce muscle spasms in the gut. Many herbs, like chamomile, blue mallow and peppermint stimulate the liver, aiding bile production and thus absorption.

Aloe Vera is a bitter herb said to have benefits for ulcers, IBS, Crohn's disease and acid indigestion. The herbs Slippery Elm and Mallow, as well as linseed and psyllium (which we're more used to think of as fibres) contain mucilage, which gives the gut a protective lining, helpful for treating inflammation or ulcerative conditions. These are now used more than bran which has somewhat gone out of fashion since studies show it can be irritating to the gut — not the result we re looking for.

BLACK COHOSH – Women's Support
(Cimicifuga racemosa)

What exactly is Black Cohosh?

Black Cohosh is a hardy perennial growing up to 9' tall. It is native to eastern North America and Native Americans have used black cohosh for centuries to treat snakebites, as mild relaxant and for 'women's concerns' hence the common names snakeroot and squawroot.

Main Functions:

A female hormonal tonic, lowers blood pressure, and nerve calming.

What does Black Cohosh actually do?

The herb's major active compound, 27–deoxyactein, possesses oestrogen-like activity, and the ability of black cohosh to selectively reduce serum concentrations of luteinising hormone (LH) even further enhance its oestrogenic effect. Black cohosh is a phytoestrogen, and it causes LH to be suppressed resulting in oestrogen remaining higher.

A Female Hormonal Tonic — The phytoestrogenic action and suppression of LH are primarily responsible for the dramatic, and clinically proven, ability of black cohosh to relieve common menopausal symptoms, such as hot flushes, depression, and vaginal dryness. Comparison studies have shown black cohosh to be far superior to HRT in reducing menopausal complains. Although research into the effect of black cohosh on bone density is currently lacking, there is justification for its use in combination with bone-building nutrients in prevention of osteoporosis. This herb may also benefit certain symptoms of premenstrual tension (*primarily oestrogen deficient forms*).

Blood Pressure Lowering - Evidence shows that black cohosh exerts a significant hypotensive effect.

Nerve Calming — Anti-anxiety and general calming effects on the nervous system have been observed. This action of black cohosh is independent of the herb's reproductive hormone effects and would further enhance any reduction in nervous tension and anxiety reported in menopausal or PMT research.

TAKE CARE
Do not use Black Cohosh when pregnant.
Do not confuse with Blue Cohosh – an entirely different plant

ECHINACEA – Immune Support
(Echinacea augustifolia)

What exactly is Echinacea?

Echinacea is a perennial growing up to 2'–5' tall. It is native to North America and Plains Americans are said to have used echinacea for more medicinal purposes than any other plant group. It is a member of the sunflower family. Its common names are Sacred Plant (by Native Americans), Black Sampsom, and Sampson root.

Main Functions

Support for the Immune System.
Prostate problems.

What does Echinacea actually do?

Echinacea can stimulate the immune system by stimulating the immune response, increasing the production of white blood cells and thus improving the body's ability to resist infections by helping to quickly eliminate infections of all kinds. Studies have shown that Echinacea even enhances the immune system in healthy people. In essence it is a natural anti-biotic.

Support for the Immune system - Echinacea stimulates the body's immune system against all infectious and inflammatory conditions specifically pathogenic infection by stimulating phagocytosis, T-cell formation, and by inhibiting the hyalurinadase enzyme secreted by bacteria to effect the breakdown of cell walls and the formation of pus. It is one of the most powerful and effective remedies against all kinds of bacterial and viral infections.

Prostate problems — Echinacea is said to be good for enlarged or weak prostate glands.

> **IMPORTANT NOTE**
> **PEOPLE WITH ANAEMIA OR VERTIGO**
> **SHOULD AVOID USING ECHINACEA**

GARLIC – Cardiovascular Support
(Allium sativun)

What exactly is Garlic?

Garlic is an onion, with the bulb made up of cloves instead of layers. Its strong-smelling pungent-tasting root is used as flavouring in cooking and for medicinal purposes. Garlic usage dates back to the Ancient Egyptian periods and civilizations have been using it for various ailments ever since.

Main functions:

Keeps heart and blood vessels healthy
Lowers harmful cholesterol in the body

What exactly does garlic do?

It is believed that the sulfur compounds and Allin/Allicin cause the beneficial actions. It is effective against bacteria that may be resistant to other antibiotics, and it stimulates the lymphatic system to throw off waster materials. Unlike other antibiotics, however, garlic does not destroy the body's beneficial flora. Instead, it has the ability to stimulate cell growth and activity, thus rejuvenating all body functions. It also fends off respiratory infections like bronchitis, pneumonia, colds and flu and infections of the urinary and digestive tract. Raw garlic crushed into salad will undoubtedly give the most benefit but can be a little anti-social.

Keeps heart and blood vessels healthy — Garlic opens up blood vessels and reduces hypertension and keeps blood pressure in the normal range, whatever the stressful situation is.

Lowers harmful cholesterol in the body — Its benefits also include lowering the harmful type of cholesterol in the body – the LDL's.

BEAR PAW GARLIC *(Alluim ursimum)* — also known as Alpine Wild Garlic is said to have more active substances than *(Allium sativun)* and therefore a potent supplement

GINGER – Digestive System support
(Zingiber officinale)

What exactly is Ginger?

Ginger is a perennial plant that grows in India, China, Mexico and several other countries. The rhizome (underground stem) is used, which contains approximately 1 – 4% volatile oils. Traditional Chinese medicine has recommended ginger for over 2,500 years.

Main functions:

Digestive system stimulant
Alleviates Nausea and Vomiting

What exactly does Ginger do?

The rich oils within the ginger-root warm and stimulate stomach and intestinal juices, encouraging complete digestion. Ginger will also benefit a congested liver with notable protective and stimulating properties. For any kind of upset stomach – ginger tea with a little lemon and honey if required should do the trick. A cup of ginger tea after meals will assist in more complete digestion, assimilation and elimination.

Digestive system stimulant – Ginger is a classic tonic for the digestive tract. Classified as an aromatic bitter, it stimulates digestion. It also keeps the intestinal muscles toned. This action eases the transport of substances through the digestive tract, lessening irritation to the intestinal walls. Ginger may protect the stomach from the damaging effect of alcohol and non-steroidal anti-inflammatory drugs (such as ibuprofen) and may help prevent ulcers. [2–4]

Nausea and Vomiting – Research is inconclusive as to how ginger acts to alleviate nausea. Ginger may act directly on the gastrointestinal system, it may affect the part of the central nervous system that causes nausea, or it may exert a dual effect in reducing nausea and vomiting. Double-blind research has shown that ginger reduces nausea after surgery. Other studies have found ginger helpful for preventing motion sickness, chemotherapy-induced nausea, and nausea of pregnancy.[5-12]

GINGKO BILOBA – Nervous System support
(Gingko Biloba)

What exactly is Gingko Biloba?

The Gingko Tree according to fossil records has existed for some 150 million years. The tree is definitely a survivor — when the atom bomb destroyed Hiroshima, the first green shoot to emerge from the blackened ashes was Gingko. Gingko's history goes back over 5,000 years in Chinese herbal medicine and is probably the planet's longest living tree.

Main functions:

Increases circulation
Nerve protection

What exactly does Gingko Biloba do?

Gingko is an adaptogen and an antioxidant. Gingko can increase circulation to the brain, the hands and the feet, improve memory and alertness and protect the heart. Recent studies in Europe have found that ginkgo helps prevent strokes by preventing the formation of blood clots. Its ability to inhibit the clumping of blood platelets is beneficial because clumps and clots contribute to heart problems, strokes and artery disease. The herb strengthens arteries in the legs and relieves pain, cramping and weakness. By increasing circulation it prevents muscular degeneration.

Increases circulation – Gingko regulates the tone and elasticity of blood vessels making the circulation more efficient. This improvement efficiently extends to both large vessels (arteries) and smaller vessels (capillaries) in the circulatory system.

Nerve protection – One of the primary protective effects of the active ingredients within the plant are their ability to inhibit a substance known as Platelet-Activating Factor (PAF) which, when released from cells, causes platelets to clump together. High amounts of PAF have a negative effect on the nervous system. Much like free radicals, higher PAF levels are also associated with aging. The active ingredients protect nerve cells in the central nervous system from damage.

BE PATIENT — It may be two weeks before you start noticing the benefits.

GINSENG – Energy and Endocrine System support
(Panax schin-seng) Korean Ginseng; (Eleutherococcus), Siberian Ginseng (Panax quinquefolium) – Wild American Ginseng

What exactly is Ginseng?

Known as 'the king of the herbs' in the Orient Ginseng is native to China. Used for over 5,000 years Ginseng is known for its rejuvenating qualities. It takes six years to mature and there are 700 species of herbs, trees and shrubs. It grows in tropical and temperate regions especially in the American tropics and the Indo-Malaysian region. Ginseng is extracted from the roots.

Main functions:

Anti-Stress herb and rejuvenation remedy.

What exactly does Ginseng do?

Ginseng stimulates the entire body to overcome stress, fatigue and weakness. There are several types of Ginseng. People over 40 should only use Red Ginseng. This is sold as Korean or Chinese ginseng. It warms up and regulates hormones and supports energy and sex drive. It is also excellent for the digestive tract. American ginseng soothes jangled nerves and regulates hormones. This ginseng is for rejuvenation and promotes a good night's sleep. American ginseng is fine for any age. Can be used continuously for up to 9 months for full effect. It is best taken with food mornings and evenings.

Siberian ginseng is altogether different coming from a different botanical plant group and is known as Eleuthero. Used to help you adapt to stress *of any kind* and maintain "balance" in your life. This herb will help you go the distance whether a sportsman or businessman and is great for travelers for reducing the unpleasant side effects of jet-lag. Its effects get better as time goes on and can be taken continually.

Anti-Stress herb - In stressful situations, the adrenal glands release corticosteroids and adrenaline, which prepare the organism for the fight or flight reaction. When these hormones are depleted, the organism reaches an exhaustive phase. Siberian Ginseng delays the exhaustive phase and allows a more economical and efficient release of these hormones.[13]

QUERCETIN — Allergy support

What exactly is Quercetin?

Quercetin belongs to a class of water-soluble plant pigments called flavonoids. It can be found in onions, apples, and black tea with smaller amounts found in leafy green vegetables and beans.

Main functions:

Anti-histamine, antioxidant and anti-inflammatory. Quercetin also protects the stomach from ulcer disease and gastric distress and strengthens capillary walls.

What exactly does Quercetin do?

Anti-histamine medication bought from a pharmacy work by pre-venting the binding of IgE and antigens to mast cells. *(refer to Immune System for fuller details)*. Quercetin on the other hand blocks histamines at the site of release by stabilising mast cells and basophils and inhibiting inflammatory enzymes and decreasing the number of leukotrienes coursing through the body. It is also said to inhibit enzymes like lipooxygenase, which are found in the inflammatory pathways that cause allergy symptoms. Quercetin has no known side effects and works quickly. When taken with other natural anti-histamines and anti-inflammatories, there are even more remarkable results.

Quercetin works in two ways. First by its anti-inflammatory properties, keeping lungs, nasal passages and eyes from welling as they normally do when allergens like pollen come into contact with the body. Secondly because Quercetin is a potent antihistamine that prevents the release of chemicals that make our nose run and our eyes water. This is achieved without the usual side effects of antihistamine drugs. It is extremely rare for Quercetin to cause side effects.

The antioxidant activities of Quercetin protects LDL cholesterol (the harmful cholesterol) from becoming damaged. Cardiologists believe that damage to LDL cholesterol is an underlying cause of heart disease.

Since flavonoids help protect and potentiate vitamin C, Quercetin is often taken with vitamin C. Quercetin is perfectly safe for children to use and a much better choice and an over the counter antihistamine.

RHODIOLA — Stress support

What exactly is Rhodiola?

Rhodiola is an adaptogenic herb that acts predominantly on the hypothalamus in a way that normalises the manner in which the body responds to stress triggers.

Main functions:

Antioxidant, anti-depressant, mental enhancer, male sexual tonic and immune supportive.

What exactly does Rhodiola do?

Antioxidant - The herb's active components are shown to be powerful antioxidants.

Anti-depressant – Rhodiola's role in aiding depression is due to various factors. Active compounds in this herb enhance the transport of serotonin precursors (tryptophan and 5–HTP) into the brain, and through an MAO/COMT inhibiting effect these compounds also reduce the degradation of mood-elevating neurotransmitters. With respect to serotonin, the studies show a 30% increase of levels in the brain. As stress accelerates the destruction of mood-boosting neuro-transmitters, the adaptogenic effects of Rhodiola would be additionally valuable.

Mental enhancer – Rhodiola intake may also boost learning and memory skills. Improvements have been shown even after 10 days treatment with Rhodiola extract.

Male Sexual tonic – Rhodiola has traditionally been used as a tonic to enhance male sexual function. Subsequent research in the field has confirmed its therapeutic effect in certain sexual dysfunction. For example, in one study involving men suffering from a weak erection and/or premature ejaculation, treatment with Rhodiola extract led to substantial improvement in sexual function.

Immune Supportive – research suggests that Rhodiola's benefits extend to the immune system – a factor that combines especially well with its adaptogenic activity. Not surprisingly, it has been reported that Rhodiola is particularly effective in aiding recovery after viral infection.

SAW PALMETTO – Prostate support
(Serenoa repens)

What exactly is Saw Palmetto?

Saw Palmetto is a dwarf palm tree native to the Atlantic coast of the United States. The active ingredient in saw palmetto is from a specific fat-soluble extract found in the tree's berries.

Main functions:

Prostate support, and general healing purposes.

What exactly does Saw Palmetto do?

One series of controlled trials showed Saw Palmetto to reduce nocturia by up to 74 per cent. The prostate is a walnut shaped male genital gland that sits at the base of the penis, right below the bladder. It surrounds the first inch of the urethra, the thin tube that carries urine to the bladder. BPH (benign prostatic hypertrophy) occurs when the prostate grows enlarged or swollen. Common symptoms include frequent urination, urinary urgency, burning while urinating and 'dribbling', all of which stem from the blockage of the bladder and urethra due to the enlarged prostate. As the bladder gets squeezed smaller and smaller, it thickens, leaving less room to store urine and causing the urgent and persistent need to urinate. Many men, usually over 40, may begin to experience problems in urinating, which can be painful and embarrassing. As men reach this age, the prostrate gland starts to grow. As it gets bigger the tube that conducts the urine out of the body gets smaller the result being the urine is very slow or comes out in little spurts resulting in having to go to the toilet more frequently, especially at night.

After the age of 50 men should consider using saw palmetto as a routine precaution, and especially if they notice any symptoms.

Choose brands that are familiar to you and are 'solvent free' and hexane-free'. Again patience is a virtue – it may take 3 – 56 weeks before you notice the benefits. Benefits include less pain, more frequency, less irritation, more control an comfort – so the wait is worth it.

ST JOHN'S WORT – Nervous System support
(Hypericum perforatum)

What exactly is St. John's Wort?

The herb St. John's Wort is found throughout North and South America, Europe and the Canary Islands, North Africa, large parts of Asia, china, Australia and New Zealand and is often described as the 'many sided' healing plant. If you hold the leaves up to the light they look perforated, hence the Latin name *'perforatum'*. These perforations are actually glands which contain volatile oil. When the flowers are squeezed between the fingers, a blood red juice emerges. Its colour comes from the main active component of St. John's Wort – hypericin.

Main functions:

Anti-depressant, anti-bacterial, nerve relaxant and mild sedative, anti-microbial, anthelmintic, inhibits infections, pain reducing, reduces bleeding, protects capillaries, and helps insomnia (especially when linked to depression).

What exactly does St. John's Wort do?

For a long time St. John's Wort was only known as 'red oil' for external use in the treatment of wounds. Its effect as a nerve medication and antidepressant when applied internally has only recently been rediscovered. Prescribed by doctors throughout Europe this is a safe, natural way to ease depression and anxiety. German medical researchers have shown the herb to be just as effective as pharmaceutical antidepressants like Prozac but without the side effects.

It is scientifically proven that depressed people have a disturbed biochemical equilibrium, which prevents the brain from operating optimally. This can lead to mental, spiritual and emotional disturbances as well as physical disturbances which fall under the heading of 'depression'. St. John's Wort affects the messenger compound dopamine, which regulates the hormone adrenaline and neurotransmitter noradrenaline. It inhibits nerve signals so that the psychic equilibrium is re-established. St. John's Wort stabilises dopamine so that the noradrenaline is not released.

Latest research also shows that St. John's Wort also has an effect on the pineal gland which, among other things, regulates the release of the hormone melatonin. When there is not enough light, for example in winter, too much melatonin may be released during the day so that the disturbed rhythm leads to sleepiness, irritability and depressive symptoms. This is the case in the typical 'winter depression'.

St. John's Wort also influences the enzyme monoamine oxydase 'MAO' (enzymes which degrade mood-elevating neurotransmitters in the brain). St. John's Wort inhibits MAO, which itself inhibits the activity of the neurotransmitter serotonin in the brain. This is an activity, which should be as free and uninhibited as possible because serotonin is a type of 'happy hormone' releasing substances that reduce pain, make on feel relaxed and allows sleep.

As opposed to anti-depressants, which require a prescription and often produce side effects, St. John's Wort can easily be bought from health food stores in capsules, juice to drink or massage oil, and side effects very seldom occur. If they do, they disappear immediately after the herb is discontinued. St. John's Wort is compatible with all other medications with the possible exception of MAO inhibitors. Avoid using the herb with MAO inhibiting or selective serotonin re-uptake inhibiting (SSRIs) drugs, unless directed by a qualified medical practitioner.

PATIENCE
Patience is needed when taking St. John's Wort for depression. It may take 3 – 4 weeks before any improvement in shown

---

REMEMBER
St. John's Wort may cause photosensitivity, especially with regular Use of high doses. Do not sunbathe or use solariums if you are taking St. John's Wort.

VALERIAN — Nervous System support
(Valeriana officinalis)

What exactly is Valerian?

Valerian is a herb grown all over Europe although most of the valerian used for medicinal extracts is cultivated. The root is used.

Main functions:

Insomnia and Anxiety

What exactly does Valerian do?

Known as the relaxing and sleep-promoting herb, it works on the brain and spinal cord and, unlike pharmaceutical drugs like Valium, has no side effects. Valerian root contains many different constituents, including essential oils that appear to contribute to the sedating properties of the herb. Central nervous system sedation is regulated by receptors in the brain known as GABA-A receptors. Valerian weakly bind to these receptors to exert a sedating action.[25] Valerian helps people deal with stress more effectively.[26]

Double blind studies have repeatedly found that valerian is more effective than placebo and as effective as standard sleep medications for people with insomnia.[27] [28] Generally valerian makes sleep more restful as well as making the transition to sleep easier but does not tend to increase total time slept according to these studies. Combining lemon balm and honey with valerian did not make it any more effective in another double blind study involving people with difficulty sleeping.[29]

Valerian is a very safe herb. It does not impair ability to drive or operate machinery, and does not lead to addiction or dependence. Valerian is not contraindicated during pregnancy or lactation, and is safe for children at half the adult dose.

A cup of Valerian tea before bedtime works wonders.

VITEX – Endocrine System support
(Vitex Agnus Castus)

What exactly is Vitex?

Chaste Tree is a member of the Verbena family, native to the Mediterranean and Central Asia. It is a shrub with finger-shaped leaves and slender violet flowers. It blooms in the summer and develops a dark brown or black berry the size of a peppercorn. The fruit has a spicy pepper like aroma and taste. The dried ripe fruits are used medicinally.

Main functions:

PMS, breast tenderness, infertility due to anovulation, menstrual problems including hypermenorrhea, poor lactation,[22] may be helpful for hot flushes, uterine fibroids, ovarian cysts and endometriosis.

What exactly does Vitex do?

Vitex or Agnus Castus as it is often called, modulates progesterone levels by increasing luteinizing hormone (LH) and decreasing follicle stimulating hormone (FSH) in the pituitary gland.[23] It also modulates prolactic secretion from the pituitary gland. Also known as chaste-berry, Vitex is one of the best-known herbs for PMS and menopausal symptoms. The liquid tincture give good results, and taken in a little warm water in the mornings can help such symptoms as mod swings, cravings, acne, excessive menstrual bleeding and irregular cycles.

A large study in Europe of 153 gynecologists working with 551 patients with premenstrual syndrome and menstrual disorders found it to be quite effective. Improvement in symptoms were found in 31.9% of patients within the first four weeks and 83.5% within 12 weeks, with 29% becoming symptom free by the end of the study. Only 11% showed no response to the treatment. About 5% reported side effects, all of them mild, with the exception of one individual who experienced heavy headaches who did not complete the treatment.[24]

Vitex has few side effects. 1–2% of patients in studies reported nausea, increased menstrual flow, acne and skin rash .

Vitex is contraindicated in pregnancy due to hormonal effects, but is used in lactation to increase milk production.

TAKE CARE
VITEX AND BLACK COHOSH HAVE *OPPOSITE* ACTIONS
USE BLACK COHOSH FOR LOW ESTROGEN LEVELS (30% of clients) AND VITEX FOR HIGH ESTROGEN (70% of clients)
THE HERB *DON QUAI* IS AN ADAPTOGEN AND CAN SAFELY BE USED SAFELY FOR EITHER HIGH OR LOW ESTROGEN LEVELS

HERBAL REMEDIES RULE NO 1
Always read the label
and follow the manufacturer's instructions exactly

HERBAL REMEDIES RULE NO 2
Results are not instantaneous –
Patience and taking the supplement on a regular basis is needed.

SUPERFOODS

There is no doubt that early physicians used food as the mainstay prescription against disease. Among these medicinal foods, cabbage was considered a 'cure all' and ancient Egyptians declared that consumption of cabbage would cure as many as 87 diseases and that consumption of onions would cure 28. Garlic was considered a holy plant. Cruciferous vegetables (cabbage and broccoli) were cultivated primarily for medicinal purposes and were used therapeutically against headache, deafness, diarrhoea, gout, and stomach disorders. The ancient Romans believed that lentils were a cure for diarrhoea and conducive to an even temper. Raisins and grapes had many medicinal uses and were incorporated into oral preparations, enemas, inhalations, and topical applications.

Superfoods are the term used to describe some of the most nutritionally concentrated foods known to man. Low on the food chain and bursting with vitality and energy they include microscopic algae, humble grasses and exotic mushrooms, some of which have been around for thousands if not millions of years. They include sprouted grains we may pass by in the supermarket like alfalfa, and ordinary foods such as mushrooms and cabbage. These foods are known as superfoods because they are packed with powerful nutritional and medicinal properties, including enzymes, pigments, vitamins, minerals and other nutrients essential for health vitality and well being.

There follows a brief description of ten superfoods. Experiment with these and other new foods for yourself, before recommending them to your clients. A recommendation is much more convincing if you have experienced the benefits for yourself.

ALFALFA
(Medicago sativa)

Main functions

Natural laxative and diuretic, cleanser especially for the liver, used for urinary tract infections, kidney, bladder and prostrate disorders.

The Chinese have used alfalfa since the sixth century to treat kidney stones, and to relieve fluid retention and swelling. It is a perennial herb that grows throughout the world in a variety of climates. Alfalfa grows to about 3 feet and has blue-violet flowers that bloom from July to September.

First discovered by the Arabs, they dubbed this valuable plant the 'father of all foods'. They fed alfalfa to their horses claiming it made the animals swift and strong. The leaves of the alfalfa plant are rich in minerals and nutrients, including calcium, magnesium, potassium and carotene (useful against both heart disease and cancer). Leaf tablets are also rich in protein, vitamins E and K. Alfalfa extract is used by food makers as a source of chlorophyll and carotene.

The leaves of this remarkable legume contain eight essential amino acids. Alfalfa is a good laxative and a natural diuretic. It is useful in the treatment of urinary tract infections and kidney, bladder and prostrate disorders. Alfalfa also alkalises and detoxifies the body, especially the liver. Promotes pituitary gland function and contains an anti-fungus agent.

Alfalfa can be bought in many different ways all of which are beneficial, but the best all round use of it is to sprout it yourself. In this way you can have fresh alfalfa sprouts every day and benefit from its many medicinal effects. Alfalfa sprouts are delicious – pack them into sandwiches and pitta breads instead or as well as lettuce.

ALGAE

With the advent of intensive farming in the West and the progression of nutrient depleted soils, there has been much interest in the benefits of blue-green micro-algae as a truly complete food form which comes from many unspoiled lakes around the world. The three main varieties that are now sold commercially as food supplements in their dried state are **Spirulina, Chlorella and Blue-Green Agae.**

Main functions:

Antioxidants, assists weight control, stimulates red blood cell formation, natural liver cleanser, aids colon irregularities, boosts the immune system, counteracts inflammatory conditions such as sore throats, ulcers, arthritis and gingivitis (gum disease), iron deficiency anaemia, depression, uplifting qualities.

Spirulina, Chlorella and Blue-Green Algae all contain a broad spectrum of vitamins, minerals and other nutrients. Their protein content is highly absorbable and they possess more chlorophyll and nucleic acids than any other plant and are abundant in enzymes. Much of the healing properties of blue-green algae are put down to their chlorophyll content. Chlorophyll is the green pigment in plants that functions to collect and store energy from the sun. Because the chlorophyll molecule is almost identical to the haemoglobin molecule in red blood cells, it has become known as "nature's blood". Like haemoglobin, chlorophyll consists of a linked series of four carbon and nitrogen containing rings (pyrrole rings). The two differ in that the centre of the ring in haemoglobin contains iron and in chlorophyll it is magnesium.

It has been shown that chlorophyll can stimulate the production of red cell formation in the blood. Foods rich in this substance have been used to treat iron deficiency anaemia with exceptional results. Chlorophyll has the added bonus of being rich in organic iron, and promotes the growth of beneficial bacteria. Other benefits of chlorophyll include its ability to cleanse the body and aid colon disorders. It also helps to speed up wound healing, boost the immune system and counteract inflammatory conditions such as sore throats, ulcers, arthritis and gingivitis (gum disease).

Spirulina is rich in vitamin B12 containing more than twice the amount found in liver. It also has 58 times more iron than raw spinach and is particularly high in beta-carotene and many other antioxidant nutrients. Spirulina also provides one of the highest sources of GLA and contains all 8 of the Essential Amino Acids making it a favourite supplement for athletes wanting to maintain lean muscle mass and a healthy muscle to fat ratio.

Spirulina is beneficial for weight control, not only because it nourishes the body so completely that it thwarts the craving for excessive food intake, but because it contains high levels of phenylalanine, an amino acid that curbs the appetite. Russian scientists have discovered that Spirulina contains thyroxin factors which may nourish the thyroid, normalise the metabolism and promote weight loss.

Chlorella can protect the liver from toxic damage by way of a substance called ethionine. Chlorella contains slightly less protein than spirulina, but it contains four times as much chlorophyll, which contributes to its powerful detoxifying properties. Its cell walls can bind to toxic substances in the body and carry them out of the system. These toxic substances not only include uranium, lead, cadmium and mercury but insecticides and pesticides. The substance ethionine is a compound that prevents the build up of fatty tissue in the liver. Chlorella possesses a greater quantity of essential fatty acids than other forms of micro-algae and about 20 per cent of these are the omega 3 variety. Being a good source of vitamin B12, iron and zinc, vegans and vegetarians, the elderly, and those recovering from illness can benefit from supplementation.

Blue-Green Algae – This algae is grown wild in the mineral rich waters of Klamath Lake in Oregon, USA. The algae contains a range of all the essential amino acids, almost identical to the balance required for human health. It is valued for its potent antioxidant properties, high levels of B12, trace minerals, and substances called sulpholipids, which have the ability to inhibit the spread of viruses.

Blue green algae can be used to alleviate depression and mental or physical sluggishness. It contains low molecular weight peptides, which are precursors of neurotransmitters, responsible for firing and calming the brain. Because of its effect on the mind, small daily dosages are recommended at first, which can then be build on over a period of several weeks.

The elderly have reported a return of mental alertness after taking blue green algae, and it has been known to arrest the degenerative process of Alzheimer's disease.

Blue green algae has also been shown to be useful in the treatment of certain neuro-stimulant addictions, such as cocaine and amphetamines. This is because it stimulates the opening of neural pathways and provides a healthy, natural energising effect. Because of its uplifting qualities, wild blue-green algae should be used with caution in those with a frail or sensitive constitution. Spirulina or Chlorella in these instances would be more appropriate. However, it can be excellent for those with a sluggish metabolism, those who are overweight or where there are signs of dietary excess.[15]

A COMPARISON BETWEEN SOME OF THE BUTRIENTS IN SPIRULINA, CHLORELLA AND BLUE GREEN ALGAE

100 gram samples (dry weight)	SPIRULINA	CHLORELLA	BLUE-GREEN ALGAE
PROTEIN	68%	55%	60%
BETA-CAROTENE	250,000 ius	55,000 ius	70,000 ius
IRON	58mg	133mg	130mg
CHLOROPHYLL	0.7–1.1%	7%	3–6%
RNA/DNA	4.5%	13%	N/A

BARLEY GRASS
(Hordeum vulgare)

Main functions:

Respiratory infections, lowers cholesterol levels, immune stimulant, natural cleanser, and stimulates blood circulation — particularly to the peripherals.

Young cereal grasses have long been recommended as a part of a cleansing and detoxifying diet but in addition they are extremely rich in vitamins, minerals, proteins and enzymes as well as containing high levels of chlorophyll, the pigment which gives all plants their green colour.

Wheat and barley, common cereal grains, start as short grasses. The plants grow slowly throughout the winter, accumulating and storing vitamins and minerals in their leaves. This grass stage lasts for about

200 days and as the plants reach their nutritional peak in the spring, they begin to form a joint which will go on to produce the stalk of grain. Once jointing occurs, the nutrient levels drop dramatically. These stored nutrients are not needed for the production of the grain so the grass is usually harvested just before jointing, using only the top three inches of the plant which is the most nutritious part. The leaves are then spray dried at low temperature and turned into tables and powders.

Barley grass is said to be the only vegetation on the earth that can supply sole nutritional support from birth to old age. Barley has served as a food staple in most cultures. The use of barley for food and medicinal purposes dates to antiquity. Agronomists place this ancient cereal grass as being cultivated as early as 7000BC. Roman gladiators ate barley for strength and stamina. In the West, it was first known for the barley grain in produces.

Barley grass is one of the richest natural sources of the enzyme superoxide dismutase (SOD). This is an antioxidant, which occurs naturally in the body and protects against free radical damage. Known as the anti-ageing enzyme, it is found in every single cell of the body and studies have shown that it can help repair damaged DNA which may help to slow down the ageing process.

Astounding amounts of vitamins and minerals are found in green barley leaves. The leaves have an ability to absorb nutrients from the soil. When barley leaves are 12–14 inches high, they contain many vitamins, minerals and proteins necessary for the human diet, plus chlorophyll. These are easily assimilated throughout the digestive tract, giving our bodies instant access to vital nutrients. These include potassium, calcium, magnesium, iron, copper, phosphorus, manganese, zinc, beta carotene, B1, B2, B6, vitamin C, folic acid, and pantothenic acid. Indeed, green barley juice contains 11 times the calcium in cows' milk, nearly 5 times the iron in spinach, 7 times the vitamin C in oranges and 80mg of vitamin B12 per hundred grams.

Barley also contains a glucan, a fiber also found in oat bran and reported to reduce cholesterol levels. The root contains the alkaloid hordenine, which stimulates peripheral blood circulation and has been used as a bronchodilator for bronchitis. Barley bran, like wheat bran may be effective in protecting against the risk of cancer.

Many health food stores sell dried barley powder to make up into a drink, or as tablets which is also an excellent way of obtaining this wonderful health food but nothing compares to the real thing. If ever you are in London a visit to Planet Organic is a must where they will prepare a 'shot' of fresh green barley grass for you to drink on the spot. Make it your first call before your shopping trip, and you will still be going strong at the end of the day!

BEE POLLEN

Main functions:

Enhances fertility, antioxidant, enhances vitality, natural tonic, strengthens the immune system, natural anti-histamine, regulates blood pressure, and assists weight loss, colitis and constipation.

Honeybees produce not only bee pollen, but also propolis, honey, royal jelly, beeswax and venom. The Bible, the Koran and ancient writings from Greece, Rome and Russia all mention and praise bee pollen as a superfood, possessing many health giving and medicinal qualities.

Bee Pollen contains the male gametes of plants found as small dust pellets in the stamen of flowers. It is gathered from pollen laden bees by a special device placed at the entrance of the hive designed to brush the material from their hind legs.

Bee Pollen has been called nature's perfect food. It is very rich in vitamins and contains almost all known minerals, trace elements, enzymes and amino acids. It contains the essence of every plant from which bees collect pollen, in combination with digestive enzymes from the bees.

Bee pollen contains broad spectrum of nutrients, including all of those required by the human body. It is made up of approximately 25% complete protein, consisting of at least 18 amino acids. This makes it a better class of protein than beef. Pollen also provides more than a dozen vitamins, 28 minerals, 11 enzymes, 14 beneficial fatty acids and 11 carbohydrates.[19]

These combinations of elements make bee pollen an excellent source of antioxidants. Research studies and clinical tests have demonstrated that bee pollen not only has an immunising effect but enhances vitality, and can counteract the effects of radiation and chemical toxins.

Used as an immune system builder, bee pollen is thought to have the ability to correct body chemistry and eliminate unhealthy conditions. It is considered to have the ability to throw off poisons and toxic materials from the body. Radiation and chemical pollutants are known as the most severe stressors to your immune system. Side effects of radiation treatment decrease the body's production of blood cells and nutrients in the blood.

Bee pollen is rapidly absorbed into the blood stream and stimulates immunological responses. It has proved beneficial for nausea, sleep disorders, and urinary and rectal disorders following radiation treatment.

Athletes often use this supplement to help increase their strength, endurance energy and speed. Bee pollen aids the body in recovering from exercise, returning breathing and heart rate to normal, and improves endurance for repeat exertion. It provides energy, stamina and strength as well as improving mental and physical reactions.

Those who do taxing mental work also can see benefits from this natural energy food. Bee pollen can relieve brain fatigue and improve alertness. This can increase your capacity for intense concentration and enable longer periods of work without becoming tired. Stress can use up vitamins quickly and bee pollen can relieve stress and anxiety by replacing essential nutrient reserves in the body.

Many people with allergies have found relief by ingesting bee pollen. It reduces the production of histamine which can cause allergic responses such as hay fever. It can strengthen the respiratory system and provide protein that can help the body build a natural defense shield against allergic responses.

Bee pollen has an effect on blood pressure and sexual function. People who suffer from low blood pressure can be subject to deficiencies in the sex glands. Pollen increases blood pressure especially when taken with kelp and may increase hormone levels and sexual strength.

Weight loss also may occur as lecithin, an ingredient in bee pollen, increases the speed calories are burned and stabilises poor metabolism. It aids in the digestive process and the assimilation of nutrients. Bee pollen may also relieve anemia, cerebral haemorrage, colitis and constipation.

CABBAGE

Main functions:

Anti-bacterial, anti-viral, heals stomach ulcers, manages oestrogen, prevents colon cancer and fights against stomach, and other cancers.

The *indoles* in cabbage, and the other cruciferous vegetables, accelerate a process in which the body deactivates or disposes of the type of oestrogen that can promote breast cancer.

Oestrogen is a known promoter of breast cancer, thus all women, but especially women with breast cancer and pre-menopausal women, should try to reduce the oestrogen circulating in their bodies, the oestrogens that may promote cancers. Cabbage and other cruciferous vegetables, such as broccoli, as well as wheat bran, have accelerated the metabolism of such oestrogen in human studies. Both foods tended to deplete body oestrogen supplies that could otherwise feed cancer. It is recommended that all women may want to try to lower circulating oestrogen by eating raw cruciferous vegetables, cabbage, broccoli, cauliflower, kale and turnips as well as wheat bran foods.

In addition cabbage contains natural anti-ulcer drugs. In the 1950's Garnett Cheney M.D., a professor of medicine at Stanford University School of Medicine showed that cabbage could help heal ulcers. He demonstrated that just over $1\frac{1}{2}$ pints (850ml) of fresh cabbage juice every day relieved pain and healed both gastric and duodenal ulcers better and faster than standard treatments did. In a test of 55 patients who drank cabbage juice, 95 per cent felt better within two to five days. X-rays and gastroscopy revealed a rapid healing of gastric ulcers in only one-quarter of the average time. The duodenal ulcers of patients fed cabbage also healed in one-third the usual time.

In a double blind-study of 45 inmates at San Quentin Prison in California, 93 per cent of the ulcers in prisoners taking cabbage juice concentrate in capsules – the equivalent of just over $1\frac{1}{2}$ pints (850ml) of fresh cabbage juice every day – were healed after three weeks. Only 32 per cent of the ulcers healed in those taking a dummy capsule. It works by seemingly strengthening the stomach lining's resistance to acid attacks. Cabbage contains gefarnate, a compound used as an anti-ulcer drug, as well as a chemical that resembles carbenoxolone, another infrequently used anti-ulcer drug. Essentially, the drugs incite cells to spin out a thin mucus barrier as a shield against acid attacks. Indeed, G B Singh, of India's Central Drug Research Institute in Lucknow, induced ulcers in guinea pigs and cured them with cabbage juice. During the healing he took extensive microscopic photos of the cell changes documenting that cabbage juice generated increased mucus activity that rejuvenated ulcerated cells leading to healing.

Another possibility is that cabbage is an antibiotic. It can destroy a variety of bacteria in test tubes, perhaps including *H.Pylori* bacteria, now implicated as a cause of ulcers.[20]

In studies, eating cabbage more than once a week cut men's colon cancer odds by 66 per cent. As little as two daily tablespoons of cooked cabbage protected against stomach cancer.

Remember what your mothers and grandmothers told you about throwing away the cabbage water? So now you know – never throw away the water but make the gravy with it or better still drink it. For best results raw cabbage, as in a coleslaw in the most beneficial, or very lightly steamed. Chinese cabbage is said to have even more beneficial properties.

HONEY

Main functions:

Anti-microbial and Anti-bacterial – stimulates the immune system, used to treat stomach ulcers, varicose and skin ulcers, wounds, burns, sore throats, acne, eczema and boils.

Honey is 'manufactured' in one of the world's most efficient factories, the beehive. Bees may travel as far as 55,000 miles and visit more than two million flowers to gather enough nectar to make just a pound of honey. It is the most popular of the bee products.

Honey is primarily composed of fructose, glucose, maltose, and water. It also contains other sugars as well as small amounts of trace enzymes, minerals, vitamins and amino acids.

Honey can both destroy harmful bacteria that could be causing digestive upset and promote beneficial bacteria in the gut.

There is no doubt that honey has healing properties. Its use can be traced back to Egyptian times. However, the therapeutic activity of honey differs according to which types of flowers the nectar has been gathered from. Honey can be made from clover, eucalyptus, and lavender to name just three. There are certain honeys that are particularly high in anti-bacterial properties, the most notably active being Manuka (or tea tree) honey from New Zealand.

Manuka honey can be effective against the *H.pylori* bacteria that is implicated in peptic ulcers. Active Manuka honey is also effective in treating bacterial gastroenteritis in infants and there is evidence that some strains of honey are prebiotic (stimulates the activity of the body's own existing good bacteria). Honey is not the only superfood that has these gut flora boosting properties — other foods include chicory, artichoke, garlic, onion, leek, asparagus, peaches and bananas.

Used topically, honey can be applied to burns, varicose and skin ulcers, wounds, acne, eczema and boils. Excellent results were found in recent clinical trials held in New Zealand when active Manuka honey was used on previously unresponsive skin ulcers and wounds.

Other research in its early stages has found that New Zealand honeys have useful levels of antioxidants with active Manuka honey having the highest of all thus used to stimulate the immune system helping the body deal with infections.

For sore throats or at the onset of a cold, honey can be taken neat or mixed with a little warm water and swallowed. A little lemon juice added to the honey will make it even more effective.

The quality of honey can vary in its potency, depending on production. It is advisable to purchase products that have not been subjected to heat treatment as part of their processing. Heating honey above hive temperature of 36° destroys many of its active ingredients and alters the nature of the sugars in the raw material. Raw, cold-pressed honey is the best to buy.

LIQUORICE
(Glycyrrhiza glabra)

Main functions:

Anti-viral, benefits respiratory tract infections — coughs, hoarseness, sore throat, bronchitis, and anti-ulcer properties.

Liquorice is a perennial herb native to southern Europe, Asia and the Mediterranean. It is extensively cultivated in Russia, Spain, Iran and India. It is one of the most popular and widely consumed herbs in the world.

Although mainly know for its flavouring in sweets, liquorice also contains many health benefits. Ancient cultures on every continent have used liquorice, the first recorded use by the Egyptians in the 3rd century BC. The Egyptians and the Greeks recognised the herb's benefits in treating coughs and lung disease. Liquorice is the second most prescribed herb in China followed by ginseng, it is suggested for treatment of the spleen, liver and kidney. The Japanese use a liquorice preparation to treat hepatitis.

The most common medical use for liquorice is for treating upper respriatory ailments including coughs, hoarseness, sore throat and bronchitis. The main constituent found in the root is glycyrrhizin. The plant also contains various sugars (to 14%), starches (30%), flavonoids, saponoids, sterols, amino acids, gums, and essential oil. Glycyrrhizin, stimulates the secretion of the adrenal cortex hormone aldosterone.

It can be as effective as codeine, and safer, when used as a cough suppressant. Rhizomes in liquorice have a high mucilage content which, when mixed with water or used in cough drops, soothes irritated mucous membranes. The herb also has an expectorant effect, which increases the secretion of the bronchial glands. Liquorice is an effective remedy for throat irritations, lung congestion and bronchitis.

Homeopathic use of liquorice for gastric irritation dates back to the first century. Today, herbal preparations are used to treat stomach and intestinal ulcers, lowers acid levels and coat the stomach wall with a protective gel. Rarely used alone, it is a common component of many herbal teas, as mild laxative, a diuretic and for flatulence. It has also been known to relieve rheumatism and arthritis, regulate low blood sugar and is effective for Addison's disease. The root extract produces mild estrogenetic effects and it has proven useful in treating symptoms of menopause regulating menstruation and relieving menstrual cramps.

The main ingredient glycyrrhizin has also been studied for it's anti-viral properties in the treatment of AIDS. In clinical trials in Japan it prevented progression of the HIV virus by inhibiting cell infection and inducing interferon activity. Glycyrrhizin also encourages the production of hormones such as hydrocortisone, which give it anti-inflammatory properties. Like cortisone, it can relieve arthritic and allergy symptoms without side effects.

The constituent glycyrrhizin is 50 times sweeter than sugar, making it a widely used ingredient in the food industry. The distinctive flavour of liquorice makes it a popular additive to baked confectionery, liqueurs, ice cream and sweets. It is also widely used in other medicines to mask bitter tastes and also to prevent pills from sticking together. Take care as some liquorice sweets are not the real thing, they may be flavoured with anise, which does not have liquorice's therapeutic effects.

MEDICINAL MUSHROOMS

Main functions:

Immune enhancement, combat viruses and bacteria, protects the body from cancer, increase energy, wards off hunger, extends longevity and promotes overall vitality and virility, lowers blood cholesterol levels, balances blood pressure and inhibits platelet aggregation (thus reducing the likelihood of heart disease).

Another line of research indicated shiitake extracts may assist in the treatment of AIDS, herpes, and other viral conditions. Shiitake may also help to prevent or treat hepatitis and other liver conditions, chronic fatigue syndrome, influenza, tuberculosis, environmental allergies, bronchial inflammation, Hodgkin's disease and stomach ulcers.

Some species of mushrooms seem to possess certain immune-enhancing properties which although scientists do not yet fully understand them, may hold potential for the treatment of cancer and other diseases. The medicinal mushrooms include Shiitake *(Lentinus edodes)*, Maitake *(Grifola frondosa)* and Reishi *(Ganoderma Lucidum)*.

Unlike blue-green algae, spirulina and chlorophyll, mushrooms lack chlorophyll which means they cannot make food from sunlight like other plants but must absorb nutrients from the surrounding medium such as soil, decaying wood and other forest waste material.

Many of our forests would not exist without mushrooms growing amongst the roots of trees. They help their hosts to obtain mineral nutrients, resist disease and survive in conditions of drought. Fungi also have an important role to play in the role of nutrient recycling. By decaying wood and other forest wastes, they release minerals and nutrients for use by a great variety of other organisms.

Shiitake Mushrooms — Studies indicate that shiitake extracts can boost the immune system and combat viruses and bacteria. Shiitake protects the body from cancer and may even shrink existing tumors, and extracts have been successfully tested in recent years in Japan as an adjunct to chemotherapy. Researchers have found that cancer patients administered shiitake have increased survival times and more positive outcomes.

Shiitake is a rich source of various vitamins and minerals, amino acids, enzymes, fiber and nucleic acid derivatives. It contains the solid plant alcohol ergosterol, which can be converted by sunlight into Vitamin D. Much of the research into shiitake has focused on its polysaccharides, especially lentinan, which are found in both the fruiting body and the mycelium. Lentinan is thought to be crucial to the mushroom's ability to inhibit cancer, primarily by stimulating certain types of white blood cells prominent in immune function rather than by directly attacking cancer cells. Shiitake's anti-viral effects may be due to its ability to induce the production of interferon in the body. The amino acid compound eritadenine may be responsible for helping to reduce blood levels of cholesterol and fats by promoting their excretion.[16][17][18]

Maitake Mushrooms - The maitake mushroom is native to northeast Japan and has been prized in Japanese herbology for hundreds of years to strengthen the body and improve overall health. Recent research indicates that it is the most potent immunostimulant of all mushrooms. The compounds contained in maitake have the capacity to not only stimulate immune function but also to inhibit tumor growth. These compounds include polysaccharides (such as Beta-glucan) and high-molecular weight sugar polymers. Polysaccharides are complex natural sugars of plant origin that typically boost the immune system. Popular herbal immune stimulants like echinacea and astralagus also contain polysaccharides. A fraction obtained from maitake called "D-fraction" has been found very effective as an anti-tumour agent when administered orally.

Reishi Mushrooms – Traditional Chinese Medicine (TCM) values Reishi as the highest ranked medicine. Among 365 species in Seng Nong's Herbal Classic, regarded as the cornerstone of TCM, the Reishi mushroom is ranked as number 1.

In China it is called Ling Chi – the Mushroom of Immortality. Recent medical research has indicated that Reishi mushrooms are useful for treating a host of diseases including hepatitis, bronchitis, bronchial asthma, coronary disease gastric ulcers, stomach ache and migraine.

With their ancient heritage, these simple, basic superfoods appear to have immense potential for human health and they may even hold the key to some of the world's most serious diseases.

SUPER SPROUTS

Main functions:

Cleansing, anti-inflammatory, rejuvenating and immune boosting.

Sprouts are a rich source of vitamins, and a clean, cheap, uncontaminated food source. Bean sprouts, mung in particular, have been grown in the Far East for thousands of years, and are mentioned in Chinese writings dated around 2939 BC. At the end of the eighteenth century, their benefits in keeping illness at bay delighted Captain Cook when not a single man died of scurvy on the three-year voyage of the Endeavour. However, limes replaced this role and the sprout was soon forgotten in Europe.

Sprouting your own seeds is a quick, easy and incredibly cheap way of providing organic, fresh food bursting with vitality. Sprouted seeds are an almost perfect food. Grown easily at home they are the richest source of naturally occurring vitamins known. A mere tablespoon of alfalfa seeds will produce about 1kg of sprouts.

Sprouted seeds are incredibly versatile and are best eaten raw in salads, sandwiches or on their own. They can also be added to hot dishes such as soups or casseroles. This should be done at the last minute to maintain their freshness and nutrient value. The larger legumes such as chickpeas and soya beans can be lightly steamed, which aids their digestibility or added to curries and stews.

Upon germination, a seed rapidly absorbs water and swells to at least twice its original size. At the same time its nutrient content changes dramatically. The husk of the seed contains the embryo, which grows into both the root and the shoot, while the endosperm and cotyledons (the two halves which you can see inside a pea, seed or bean) become the food supply for the growing plant. During sprouting the content and activity of enzymes increase converting starch into simple sugars, protein into amino acids and fats into fatty acids. These processes in effect pre-digest the seed, making it much easier for us to break down and absorb. This is the reason why many sprouted grains and legumes are less likely to cause the allergic reactions that their non-sprouted counterparts can trigger.

The vitamin content of a sprout is particularly significant. Sprouted mung beans contain as much as 120mg of vitamin C per 100g compared with oranges, which have around 53mg. It has also been shown that the amount of B vitamins rise as a seed sprouts. The vitamin B2 content in an oat grain multiplies by 1300 per cent as soon as the seed germinates, although some Bs do not increase until the small plant grows leaves and starts to photosynthesise. Whether sprouts contain vitamin B12 appears to be undecided, although most sprouted cereals are said to possess trace amounts. The fat-soluble vitamins A D and E are also present. Minerals, which are in abundant supply, combine with amino acids to form 'chelates'. These significantly increase their uptake and use in the body. While the protein content in vegetables is not significant, sprouts are an exception. A bean or seed's protein value actually diminishes as it germinates yet a sprout is still a valid source as it builds new protein from stored nutrients within the seed.

Soya sprouts are the only ones to contain all eight essential amino acids. For people who follow a diet of food combining i.e. not mixing high protein foods with starch, sprouts bring an added bonus of being a 'neutral' so that they can be eaten with either.

Because they contain an excellent balance of amino acids, fatty acids and natural sugars, plus a high content of minerals, sprouts are capable of sustaining life on their own, provided several kinds are eaten together. They are also the cheapest form of foods around. In an age when most vegetables and fruits are grown on artificially fertilised soils and treated with hormones, DDT, fungicides, insecticides, preservatives and all manner of other chemicals, home-grown sprouts emerge as unadulterated, fresh, unpolluted and marvelous tasting food grown in just a few days.

Common seeds for sprouting are alfalfa, mung beans, aduki beans, wheat, barley, fenugreek, lentils, mustard, oats, pumpkin seeds, sesame seeds, sunflower seeds and soya beans.

Most supermarkets now sell ready sprouted seeds. Try a few different ones in salads and as additions to your sandwiches and then experiment and try sprouting your own.

HOW TO SPROUT

Small commercial sprouters are available in health food stores and usually comprise of four small trays stacked upon each other with a selection of seeds and beans and a set of instructions — which make ideal unusual presents. Alternatively, you can use a standard seed tray, a colander or sieve.

1. Place a handful of your selected seeds or beans in a bowel, cover with cold water and leave them to soak overnight. Most seeds will expand up to eight times their size so be generous with the water and totally submerge them.

2. The following morning, drain off the water, rinse well and lay the seeds in the base of the sprouter.

3. Either leave on the window sill (this is what I do) or place in an airing cupboard. The seeds need to be rinsed thoroughly at least once a day, preferably twice.

4. Continue to rinse the seeds daily until ready to harvest. After about three to five days you should have a crop of sprouts. Once they are the right size for eating, give them one final rinse and store them in the fridge to stop them from growing any further.

SPROUT HARVESTING TIMES

SEED/SPROUT	HARVEST TIME IN DAYS
Alfalfa	5–7
Aduki beans	4–6
Barley	3–4
Chickpeas	4
Fenugreek	4–5
Flageolet beans	3–5
Green lentils	3–5
Green peas	3–5
Mung beans	2–3
Radish	4–5
Rye	3–5
Soya beans	3–6
Sunflower seeds	4–6
Wheat	2–4

YOGHURT
PROBIOTICS and PREBIOTICS

Main functions:

Maintains a healthy digestive tract restoring total health to the ecology of our gasto-intestinal systems, supports the immune system, guards against cancer, combats yeast overgrowth and fungal infections such as Candida Albicans, prevents constipation, diarrhoea, flatulence and boating, protects against osteoporosis and rheumatoid arthritis, overcomes skin problems, lowers cholesterol levels and enhances nutritional status.

No book on nutrition or indeed a chapter on superfoods could be complete without mention of probiotics. Probiotics means 'for life' the opposite of antibiotics meaning 'against life'. When we take even one course of antibiotics, the harmful bacteria in our intestines are destroyed together with the beneficial bacteria resulting in a suppressed immune system. Of all the superfoods mentioned thus far, the probiotics I feel must take priority place. The roles they play in our bodies are quite amazing.

At the turn of the century a scientist named Elie Metchnikoff proposed that yogurt was the elixir of life because it contained a strain of bacteria known as *Lactobacillus* that purportedly cleared the large intestine of toxins. We now know that two particular species of probiotics, *Lactobacillus bulgaricus* and *Streptococcus thermophilus,* are the primary cultures in yogurt, and they make this dairy treat a supremely healthy food by combating certain bad bacteria and improving lactose tolerance. These two strains work together and combine their unique powers to defend the gut from potentially harmful bacteria.[21.]

Yoghurt is an ancient wonder food, strongly antibacterial and anticancer. 8oz (225g) taken on a daily basis can boost the immune function by stimulating production of gamma interferon. As well as the vitally important beneficial culture yoghurt contains, it is also a good source of absorbable calcium.

It often comes as a surprise for us to learn that the thousands of billions of bacteria living in the human gastro-intestinal tract weigh an amazing $1\frac{1}{2}$ kilos.

There have now been thousands of studies confirming that probiotics are indispensable in keeping us healthy by cleansing our intestines of excess pathogens, thus preventing allergies, yeast infections, diarrhoea, gas, bloating, and digestive problems.

The good flora also manufacture B-vitamins, such as biotin, B3, B6 and folic acid and by providing the enzyme lactase they enhance, and indeed allow, the digestion of milk-based foods, and the vital calcium which they contain, for people who cannot otherwise digest milk. They help considerably to enhance bowel function. Where bowel bacteria are absent, the function of peristalsis is impaired, and the amount of time it takes for food to pass completely through the system is much increased. The beneficial bacterial also act as anti-carcinogenic (anti-cancer) factors with powerful anti-tumour potentials.

Problems usually begin after a course of antibiotics when this beneficial bacteria is killed and not replaced. This good flora needs to be replaced after **every** course of antibiotics we take. Probiotics is all about the use of specially cultured friendly bacteria and yoghurt is one way of getting some of this good flora back into your system. Unfortunately it is impossible to know exactly how many live cultures are in the yoghurt you are eating and they may only provide a couple of hundred bacteria per pot. This is fine if you are just keeping 'topped-up' with friendly bacteria, but if you have been on a course of antibiotics, and especially if you have had concurrent courses of antibiotics, you need to replace the billions of destroyed bacteria as soon as possible. These need to come in the form of a good supplement. Always choose probiotics from human origin – and follow storage instructions carefully. Once opened the probiotics need to be refrigerated.

Many babies and children are given multiple courses of antibiotics, some even before they are one year old, suppressing an immature immune system. Antibiotics can be life saving but whenever they are used, you should always follow up with a course of probiotics. Children's formulas are available from all good health food stores.

PREBIOTICS

Probiotics and Prebiotics work in different ways to achieve the same end – keeping numbers of good bacteria up so that they outweigh pathogenic bacteria. Probiotics deliver 'ready made' good bacteria to the body whereas prebiotics stimulate the activity of the body's own existing good bacteria. Each of us carries $1\frac{1}{2}$kg of bacteria in our body of which 95% are beneficial. If the balance of these 'flora' changes 'gut dysbiosis' results and digestive disorders, stomach upsets, food poisoning and worse can arise. Numerous clinical trails show the benefits of probiotics and prebiotics in aiding digestion, stimulating gastrointestinal immunity, and relieving IBS symptoms.

Fructo-Oligosaccharides (FOS)

Work with prebiotics arose of the shortcomings of probotiics (acidophilus).

The prebiotic concept is that substrates such as FOS (a form of soluble-fibre) are ingested which favour the growth of beneficial bacteria so that the numbers or metabolic processes of harmful micro-organisms, such as Candida albicans are suppressed.

Researchers now agree that the definition of a prebiotic is a non-digestible food ingredient that beneficially affects the host by selectively stimulating the growth and/or activity of one or more of a limited number of bacteria in the colon to improve the host's health. FOS cannot diffuse across the gut mucosa and it resists being broken down by brush border enzymes. Subsequently, FOS provide energy for friendly bacterial growth.

It is through the fermentation of FOS that the short chain fatty acids such as butyric acid are produced which act as nutritive compounds for the cells that line the gasro-intestinal tract.

Fructo-Oligosaccharides can be purchased from any health food store.

PART II   BODY SYSTEMS

THE CARDIOVASCULAR SYSTEM

What is the Cardiovascular System?

The cardiovascular (circulatory) system is the body's transport system and comprises the heart, the arteries, the veins and the capillary network of arterioles and venules. The capillary network of the human body consists of over 62,000 miles of blood vessels through which our blood travels.

What does the Cardiovascular do?

Responsible for continuously pumping the blood around the body.

Main functions:

The main functions of the blood are — protection, equilibrium, clotting and transport.

Protection — Blood offers protection against foreign microbes and toxins which are destroyed by certain white blood cells that are phagocytic (engulfing) in their actions, or specialised proteins such as antibodies, interferon and complement. White blood cells are collectively called leucocytes and they play a major role in combating disease and fighting infection.

Equilibrium — Blood also regulates normal body temperature. It does this by absorbing large quantities of heat produced in the liver and the muscles. This is then transported around the body to help to maintain a constant internal temperature. The blood also helps to regulate the body's pH balance. These two actions are collectively known as homeostasis.

Clotting — Blood protects against blood loss through the clotting mechanism. Specialised red blood cells called platelets clot to prevent blood getting out and bacteria getting in.

Transport — The blood is responsible for transporting many substances around the body.

Oxygen is carried from the lungs to the cells of the body in red blood cells. It also carries carbon dioxide from the cells to the lungs, nutrients from the gastrointestinal tract to the cells, waste products from cells, hormones from endocrine glands to the cells and heat from various cells.

CARDIOVASCULAR RULE NO 1
We only have one heart.   Take care of it.

Cardiovascular disease is the number one killer in Great Britain, and there are many risk factors associated with it most of which can be managed, but some with cannot. The ageing process and hereditary predisposition are risk factors that cannot be altered. Until the age of fifty men are at grater risk than women of developing heart disease though once a woman enters menopause, her risk triples.[205]

High cholesterol levels immediately spring to mind when you think of the cardiovascular system, and many people with cardiovascular disease do have elevated cholesterol levels[206] and although cholesterol has received some bad press over the years, it isn't all bad – there is a good side to cholesterol as well. It is a constituent of cell membranes, is a precursor of bile acids and steroid hormones and vitamin D, the sunshine vitamin, also comes from cholesterol.

Homocysteine, on the other hand, is something we should be concerned about. Often cholesterol has taken the blame for heart disease when homocysteine may have been the culprit.

HOMOCYSTEINE
Having a high level of homocysteine in the blood is as great a risk factor for cardiovascular disease as smoking or having a high blood

cholesterol level. Homocysteine is made from protein in the diet. The amino acid methionine is converted into homocysteine in the body and provided you have enough vitamin B6, B12 and folic acid, the body will convert it into cystanthionine. We now know that homocysteine is very toxic and can cause the initial damage to the artery wall that starts the whole process of cardiovascular disease. There has been much research confirming that homocysteine has a role to play in cardiovascular disease and that cholesterol, in its antioxidant capacity, and in an attempt to repair the initial damage caused by the homocysteine, builds up inside the scarred arteries. This can lead to fatal blockages, and the cholesterol may then take the blame for the initial damage caused by the homocysteine.

Homocysteine levels rise with age and women have, on average 20 per cent lower levels than men until the menopause, and then the levels between the sexes are more or less equal.

Those most at risk of high homocysteine levels are those that consume a high protein diet with a poor dietary status of B6, B12 and folic acid. High homocysteine levels have been identified as an independent risk factor for coronary heart disease.[207]

Clients should be advised that if they are concerned about high cholesterol levels they should also be aware of the homocysteine connection. Tests are available to evaluate homocysteine levels, which can be measured by a blood test. (*See Appendix 1*).

Dietary influences affecting the cardiovascular system

A high meat and dairy diet accompanied with a low fiber diet are the main culprits as far as the cardiovascular system is concerned. There has been insurmountable evidence showing that people on a low animal fat and high fiber diet have less heart disease than others who restrict animal fats and dairy food in their diet. However, nothing is that simple. Fat plays a vital part of our diet, and essential fatty acids need to be ingested every day so the type of fats we choose is important. We should remember the title of Udo Erasmus' book 'Fats that Heal and Fats that Kill' – a very true statement indeed. Heart disease however, is not about diet alone, it is the result of total lifestyle habits.

COMMON DISORDERS
ANGINA

There are three main types of angina. The first is called stable angina. This type of chest pain comes on during exercise and is both common and predictable. Stable angina is associated with atherosclerosis. A second type, called variant angina, can occur at rest or during exercise. This type is primarily due to sudden coronary artery spasm, though atherosclerosis may also be a component. The third, most severe type is called unstable angina. It occurs with no predictability and can quickly lead to a heart attack. Anyone who has significant or new chest pain or a worsening of previously mild angina must seek medical assistance immediately.

It is caused by an insufficient supply of blood to the walls of the heart, which in turn induces oxygen starvation. The serious symptoms do not appear all at once but increasing instances of acute heart cramps accompanied by a feeling of tightness across the chest called cardiac insufficiency should be a warning that immediate action should be taken. Refer clients to their GP if they complain of any type of chest pain.

From an holistic point of view, relieving constipation, encouraging proper bowel function and ensuring the elimination of all waste materials is important for anyone with angina.

Cigarette smoking causes damage to the coronary arteries and, in this way can contribute to angina. Stopping smoking is the most important lifestyle change anyone can do who has angina. Smoking has also been shown to reduce the effectiveness of treatment of angina.[80] Secondhand smoke (cadmium) should also be avoided.

Increasing physical exercise has been clearly demonstrated to reduce symptoms of angina as well as to relieve the underlying causes. One study found that ten minutes intense daily exercise was as effective as beta-blocker drugs in one group of patients with angina. However, anyone with a heart condition including angina or anyone over the age of forty should consult a doctor before beginning an exercise plan.

Coffee should be avoided as drinking 5 cups or more a day has been shown to increase the risk of angina.

Carnitine is an amino acid important for transporting fats that can be turned into energy in the heart. Several studies using one gram carnitine two to three times per day show improvement in heart function and reduced symptoms in patients with angina.[81] [82] [83]

Co-Qo10 also contributes to the energy making mechanisms of the heart. Angina patients given 150mg of Co-Q-10 experienced greater ability to exercise without problems.[84] This has been confirmed by independent investigations.[85]

Low levels of antioxidant vitamins in the blood, particularly vitamin E, are associated with greater rates of angina.[86] This is true even when smoking and other risk factors are taken into account. Early, short-term studies using 300ius per day of vitamin E could not find a beneficial action on angina.[87] However, a later study supplementing small doses of vitamin E (50ius per day) for longer periods of time showed a minor benefit.[124]

Fish oil, which contains the beneficial fatty acids known as EPA and DHA, has been used in the treatment of angina. In some studies, 3 grams or more of fish oil three times per day (providing a total of about 3 grams of EPA and 2 grams of DHA) have reduced chest pains as well as the need for nitroglycerin, a common medication used to treat angina.[88] If fish oil is supplemented, vitamin E should be taken with it, as vitamin E may protect the fragile oil against free radical damage.[124] Those affected by variant angina have been found to have the greatest deficiency of vitamin E compared with other angina patients.[125]

RECOMMENDATIONS FOR ANGINA

DIET	A high fibre, unrefined carbohydrate diet providing well balanced meals containing all of the main food groups.
INCREASE	Cold water fish, plenty of fruits and raw or lightly steamed vegetables, onions, sunflower seeds and seed sprouts.
DECREASE	Coffee, salt, alcohol, coffee, sugar, refined grains, hydrogenated fats, dairy products, fried foods, red meat.
SUPERFOODS	Medicinal mushrooms, avocados, hazelnuts and almonds.
SUPPLEMENTS	Carnitine, Co-Q-10 Anti-oxidant complex containing Vitamins A, C, E and Selenium.
HERBALS	Garlic, preferably raw with food or a supplement.
LIFESTYLE CHANGES	Stop smoking. Gentle exercise – daily walking recommended – no less than 10 minutes

ARTERIOSCLEROSIS & ATHEROSCLEROSIS

Arteriosclerosis is a degenerative change in the arterial walls, affecting first the middle and later the inner layers, and resulting in loss of elasticity and possible calcification. Commonly referred to as hardening of the arteries. [102]

Atherosclerosis is a degenerative change in the arterial walls which principally affects the larger arteries such as the aorta, coronary, and cerebral vessels. More commonly referred to as a narrowing of the arteries.

The most important dietary changes for protecting the arteries from atherosclerosis include avoiding meat and dairy fat, increasing fiber and avoiding foods that contain trans-fatty acids (margarine, some vegetable oils, and many processed foods containing vegetable oils). The fibers most linked to the reduction of cholesterol levels are found in oats, psyllium seeds, and fruit (pectin). Leading researchers have recently begun to view the evidence linking trans-fatty acids to markers for heart disease as 'unequivocal.'[240]

It has been shown that foods that contain high amounts of cholesterol, mostly egg yolks, can induce atherosclerosis, so it may make sense to reduce intake of egg yolks. However, eating eggs does not increase serum cholesterol as much as eating saturated fat, and eggs may not increase serum cholesterol at all if the overall diet is low in fat. A decrease in atherosclerosis resulting from a pure vegetarian diet, meaning no meat, poultry, dairy or eggs, combined with exercise and stress reduction has been proven by medical research.[241]

Many experts agree that LDL – low-density lipoproteins – the harmful cholesterol, triggers atherosclerosis only when reactive molecules called free radicals have damaged it. There are several antioxidant supplements that protect LDL.

Vitamin E is an antioxidant that serves to protect LDL from oxidative damage and has been linked to prevention of heart disease in double blind research. Many nutritional therapists recommend 400 — 800ius of vitamin E per day to lower the risk of atherosclerosis and heart attacks.

Other studies have shown that people who consume more selenium and quercetin from their diet have a lower risk from heart disease. Quercetin, a bioflavonoid, also protects from LDL damage and can be found in apples, onions, black tea, and as a supplement. In some studies dietary amounts linked to protection from heart disease are as low as 35mg per day.

Preliminary research shows that chrondroitin sulfate may prevent atherosclerosis in animals and humans and may also prevent heart attacks in people who already have atherosclerosis. However, further research is needed to determine the value of chrondroitin sulfate supplements for preventing or treating atherosclerosis.

Reservatrol, found primarily red wine, is a naturally occurring antioxidant that decreases the 'stickiness' of blood platelets and may help blood vessels remain open and flexible. As reservatrol is now available in supplement form, there is no need for that one glass of beneficial red wine any more! The supplement will give you the reservatrol without the alcohol.

Several herbs have been shown in research to lower lipid levels. Of these, psyllium has the most consistent backing from multiple double blind trials showing lower cholesterol and triglyceride levels.[242]

Garlic has also been shown to prevent excessive platelet adhesion in humans. Allicin often considered the main active component of garlic is not alone in this action. The constituent known as ajoene has also shown beneficial effects on platelets. Garlic has also lowered cholesterol levels in double blind research.

Ginkgo Biloba may reduce the risk of atherosclerosis by interfering with a chemical the body sometimes makes in excess called platelet activating factor (PAF).[243] PAF stimulates platelets to stick together too much; ginkgo stops this from happening. Ginkgo also increases blood circulation both to the head and to the arms and legs.

Garlic and ginkgo together, also decrease excessive blood coagulation. Both have been shown in double blind or single blind studies to decrease the overactive coagulation of blood that may contribute to atherosclerosis.

CARDIOVASCULAR RULE NO 2
The heart is a muscle like any other – it needs exercise!

REMEMBER
BRANCHED CHAIN AMINO ACIDS
The branch chain amino acids, valine, leucine and isoleucine protect all muscles, including the heart
and actually makes exercise seem more enjoyable by reducing the feeling of fatigue.

RECOMMENDATIONS FOR ARTERIOSCLEROSIS

DIET	A diet consisting of brown rice, soft white cheese (quark) and salads can have fantastic results if adhered to consistently. Rice bran influences the regeneration of the arteries. Iodine rich foods can be taken as seasonings or salts. Low animal fat and dairy recommended together with a high fiber diet.
INCREASE	Oily fish — sardines, salmon, herring, tuna and mackerel with plenty of fruits and raw or lightly steamed vegetables, onions, nuts and seeds.
DECREASE	Salt, alcohol, coffee, sugar, refined grains, hydrogenated fats, dairy products, fried foods and red meat.
SUPERFOODS	Olive oil, strawberries, avocados, hazelnuts and almonds.
SUPPLEMENTS	Vitamin E alone or an antioxidant complex containing vitamins A, C, E and Selenium. Folic Acid. Lecithin granules and Psyllium seeds or husks.
HERBALS	Garlic, preferably raw in salads or as a supplement. Ginkgo Biloba.
LIFESTYLE CHANGES	Gentle daily exercise, swimming is ideal.

CHILBLAINS

Red/blue skin patches that hurt at every movement are known as chilblains. They mainly effect hands and feet and are caused by prolonged exposure to severe cold. Chilblains are a circulatory disorder and can easily be prevented.

The herb Ginkgo Biloba can help with a variety of circulatory problems from strokes to varicose veins, and is a good choice for chilblain sufferers.

Gingko Biloba, is an excellent herb, but can take a few months to 'kick-in'. In the meantime you will want to do something about your chilblains. This is one condition where you can use an Aromatherapy essential oil neat. For almost instant relief from chilblains, apply 1 drop of neat geranium oil to the affected area for two or three days, after which a massage oil can be used. Blend 10mls of Sweet Almond base oil into 3 drops geranium, 1 drop Lavender and 1 drop Rosemary. Massaging daily, leaving the oil on the skin, will quickly alleviate chilblain symptoms. At night massage the oil into the affected area and wear cotton socks or gloves to sleep in will also be of benefit.

RECOMMENDATIONS FOR CHILBLANES

DIET	A whole food approach to food where quality is more important than quantity. Plenty of fruits and vegetables, low-fat protein, and plenty of water.
INCREASE	All fruits and vegetables. Oily fish – sardines salmon, herring, tuna and mackerel.
DECREASE	Everything refined – especially white bread and flour, confectionery, and alcohol.
SUPERFOODS	Manuka honey, which can be applied directly to chilblains and lightly bandaged for a few hours. Also to eat together with Alfalfa, Algae, Medicinal mushrooms, and Bee Pollen.
SUPPLEMENTS HERBALS	Multivitamin and mineral complex. Ginkgo Biloba.
LIFESTYLE CHANGES	When coming in from the cold, do not stand in front of a fire, chilblains do not like sudden changes in temperature. Keep feet and legs well covered with natural fibers.

CHOLESTEROL (High) (Hypercholesterolemia)

Although it is by no means the only major risk factor, elevated serum cholesterol is clearly associated with a high risk of heart disease.

There are many dietary, lifestyle and supplement changes that can be of great benefit for this condition.

Usually you hear about foods you should avoid when you're trying to not raise your cholesterol such as eggs, red meat, cheeses and fried foods. There are, however, also foods known to *lower* your cholesterol levels. However, by eating these cholesterol-lowering foods, does not mean that you can indulge in the foods that are said to increase levels. The cholesterol-lowering foods are oat bran, cooked beans, carrots, olive oil and soy.

> ## TOP FIVE CHOLESTEROL LOWERING FOODS
> ### Oat Bran, Cooked Beans, Carrots, Olive Oil and Soy

Oat bran is a rich source of soluble fiber, which has been shown to help reduce cholesterol levels. Cooked beans, such as pinto and kidney are another great source of soluble fiber as well as being an inexpensive and versatile food source. Carrots on the other hand, are not a good source of soluble fiber, but a recent study showed that one raw carrot a day at breakfast could lower total cholesterol by as much as 11 per cent. Carrots contain insoluble fiber, which aids in normal bowel function by assisting to flush dietary cholesterol more quickly from the body. Olive oil is high in monounsaturated fatty acids, which has been shown to help manage cholesterol when part of a low-fat, low-cholesterol diet. This oil should replace more saturated fats in the diet like butter and margarine whenever possible, if trying to reduce cholesterol levels. Lastly, soy – found in tofu, tempeh, soymilk, roasted soy nuts and more, can help reduce cholesterol levels in the body. The higher your cholesterol the more soy will help bring your levels to where they should be, but if you already have a healthy cholesterol level, then soy will have no effect.

> ## REMEMBER
> These top five cholesterol-lowering foods will only be effective if you make them part of a diet that gets no more than 30 per cent of its total calories from fat and less than 7 per cent from saturated fatty acids.

Eating fish has been reported to increase HDL, the beneficial cholesterol[172] and is linked to a reduction in heart disease in most studies undertaken.[173] Fish contains very little saturated fat, and fish oil contains EPA and DHA, omega-3 oils that protect against heart disease.

Vegetarians have lower cholesterol[174] and less heart disease[175] than meat eaters, in principal because they avoid animal fat. Vegans (people who eat no meat, dairy, or eggs) have the lowest cholesterol levels,[176] and going on such a diet has reversed heart disease.[177]

Like cholesterol, egg consumption still remains a controversial issue. Many nutritional therapists advise that eggs are safe to eat provided they are boiled, poached or baked, and whilst eggs cooked in this way are undoubtedly safer than eggs that are scrambled or fried, care must be taken over egg consumption. It is often said that eggs are safe if the rest of the diet is low in fat, however, egg consumption does not appear to be totally safe, even for people consuming a low fat diet. When cholesterol from eggs is cooked or exposed to air, it oxidizes. Oxidised cholesterol is linked to increased heart disease[178] and eating eggs also makes LDL cholesterol more susceptible to damage, another change linked to heart disease.[179] Moreover, egg eaters are more likely to die from heart disease even when serum cholesterol levels are not elevated.[180] Therefore the idea that egg consumption is unrelated to heart disease, a position taken by many nutritional therapists and doctors of natural medicine, is not supported by most scientific evidence. My own recommendations to clients are a maximum of two free-range eggs per week, boiled, poached or baked.

There have been many studies that show chromium supplementation has reduced LDL cholesterol and increased HDL cholesterol in human studies.[181] [182] [183] Brewer's yeast, which contains readily absorbable chromium, also lowers cholesterol levels, and people with higher blood levels of chromium appear to be at a lower risk of heart disease. A reasonable and safe intake of supplemental chromium is 200mcg per day. People wishing to use brewer's yeast as a source of chromium should look for products specifically labeled 'from the brewing process' or 'brewer's yeast' because most yeast found in health food stores is not brewer's yeast and does not contain chromium. Optimally, true brewer's yeast contains up to 60mcg of chromium per tablespoon, and a reasonable intake is two tablespoons per day.

There have also been many studies showing favourable results with garlic, wild yam, and psyllium. In addition, artichoke has moderately lowered cholesterol and triglycerides in some reports.

RECOMMENDATIONS FOR HIGH CHOLESTEROL

DIET	A whole food approach to food where quality is more important than quantity. Plenty of fruits, vegetables, nuts and seeds with adequate essential fatty acids, low-fat protein, and plenty of water.
INCREASE	One raw carrot daily with breakfast, olive oil, soy, oat bran and cooked beans. Oily fish – sardines salmon, herring, tuna and mackerel to be eaten at least three times a week.
DECREASE	Red meat, eggs, hard cheese, fried foods and sugar
SUPERFOODS	Alfalfa, Barley Grass, Chlorophyll, Medicinal Mushrooms, Super Sprouts and low-fat bio-yoghurt.
SUPPLEMENTS	A multivitamin and mineral containing at least 50mgs of the B-complex group of vitamins. 600ius of Vitamin E daily 500mg Vitamin C daily Chromium in the form of Brewer's Yeast. Flax seed fiber
HERBALS	Black cohosh and garlic
LIFESTYLE CHANGES	Regular gentle exercise Giving up smoking would be of great benefit.

CARDIOVASCULAR RULE NO 3
Supplementing vitamins E and C effectively
halves the risk of ever having a heart attack!

HAEMORRHOIDS

Haemorrhoids are enlarged raised veins in the anus or rectum and are commonly known as piles. They are often associated with chronic constipation in the dense network of blood vessels that run through the intestinal lining, but can also be linked to diarrhoea.[184]

When the stool in the rectum becomes hard and accumulates there, the blood vessels become stretched. The resulting obstruction causes the walls of the vessels in the anal canal to become dilated, turning them into varicose veins. Sometimes, the pressure needed to force out hard stools makes the veins in the thin membranes rupture; making the haemorrhoids bleed. At the time of evacuation, light coloured blood may be noticed on the stool. If this condition is not remedied, the tissues will become inflamed and hard, resulting in piles. Hard stools can push the piles outwards so they hang outside the anus; these can sometimes enlarge to the size of a plum.

The first action to be taken is that of curing the constipation. Only when the constipation has been remedied you can concentrate on the haemorrhoids, as constipation may worsen haemorrhoid symptoms.

An excellent herbal product is psyllium seeds. Two teaspoons of the seeds or 1 teaspoon of the husks once or twice a day with water should be of benefit. Another herb used in the treatment of haemorrhoids is witch hazel, which is topically applied to haemorrhoids three to four times daily in an ointment base.

Fiber is undoubtedly an important aspect with regard to the treatment of haemorrhoids. Countries with high fiber intakes have a very low incidence of haemorrhoids. Insoluble fiber – the kind found primarily in whole grains and vegetables – increases the bulk of the stool. Drinking water with a high-fiber meal or supplement results in softer, bulkier stools, which can move through the large colon more easily.

RECOMMENDATIONS FOR HAEMORRHOIDS

DIET	A high-fiber, whole grain approach to bread must be taken with plenty of fresh fruit and raw vegetables.
INCREASE:	Rice bran Fruits and vegetables, prunes, figs, and dates Lots of fluids.
DECREASE	Alcohol, all refined foods, all stimulants like coffee and tea.
SUPERFOODS	Barley Grass, Spirulina.
SUPPLEMENTS	A multivitamin and mineral containing at least 50mgs of the B-complex group of vitamins.
HERBALS	Cayenne, Ginkgo Biloba, Psyllium seeds or husks, Witch hazel, A tea made from stinging nettles is also beneficial.
LIFESTYLE CHANGES	Abdominal exercises. Keep off your feet as often as possible. Cold water bathing each morning to the anus is also recommended.

HYPERTENSION

Hypertension is a medical term used to describe high blood pressure — a condition with many causes but which cannot be attributed to any one single cause.

Symptoms of high blood pressure are headache, dizziness, nervousness, irritability, low energy, fatigue, and insomnia. In most cases of hypertension we find that increased peripheral resistance (narrowing of the blood vessels, especially the small arteries) is the primary cause. Another accepted cause of high blood pressure is narrowing of the blood vessels due to cholesterol and other fatty molecules.[101]

It is estimated that 85 per cent of all cases of high blood pressure are both treatable and preventable without drugs. Diet remains the most single most important factor in controlling high blood pressure. People with mild to moderate high blood pressure should work with a nutritional therapist or a nutritionally oriented doctor to help reduce blood pressure using diet alone. However, people with extremely high blood pressure (malignant hypertension) or rapidly worsening blood pressure (accelerated hypertension) almost always require treatment with conventional medicine.

Vegetarian diets have been reported to significantly lower blood pressure.[168] This occurs partly because fruits and vegetables contain potassium – a known blood pressure-lowering mineral. The well known study *Dietary Approaches to Stop Hypertension (DASH)* increased intake of fruits and vegetables (and therefore fiber) and reduced cholesterol and dairy fat which led to large reductions in blood pressure in just eight weeks.[169]

There are many supplements that may significantly assist in lowering high blood pressure. Vitamin C plays an important role in maintaining the health of arteries and a review of vitamin C research reported that most studies linked increased blood and dietary levels of this vitamin to reduced blood pressure. The omega-3 fatty acids found in fish oil have also been found to lower blood pressure as has C-Q-10, which has shown to significantly lower blood pressure. There are also many studies to show that magnesium supplements – typically 350–500mg per day to be beneficial. Magnesium appears to be particularly effective in people who are taking *potassium depleting diuretics*.[170] Potassium depleting diuretics also deplete magnesium, so the drop in blood pressure resulting from magnesium supplementation in people taking these drugs may result from overcoming a mild magnesium deficiency.

Smoking is particularly harmful for people with hypertension.[171] The combination of hypertension and smoking greatly increases the chances of heart disease. People with high blood pressure should make stopping smoking a major priority.

As with conventional drugs, the use of natural substances sometimes controls blood pressure if taken consistently but does not lead to a cure for high blood pressure. Thus someone whose blood pressure is successfully reduced by weight loss, avoidance of saturated fats and increased intake of fruits and vegetables would need to maintain these changes *permanently* in order to maintain control of blood pressure.

RECOMMENDATIONS FOR HYPERTENSION

DIET	A low fat, high fibre diet with plenty of salads and fruits.
INCREASE	Dietary fiber, fruits and all vegetables.
DECREASE	Animal fats, saturated fats, salt in cooking and on food, caffeine and alcohol.
SUPERFOODS	Flaxseed, Super Sprouts, Medicinal Mushrooms and Bee Pollen.
SUPPLEMENTS	Flaxseed fiber. A Multivitamin and mineral complex with additional 1g of vitamin C. Vitamin E. Fish Oils and Co-Q-10.
HERBALS	Black cohosh, Garlic, Ginger, Siberian Ginseng.
LIFESTYLE CHANGES	Weight loss and an increase in regular gentle exercise. Do not add salt to your food. Give up smoking.

HYPOTENSION

Hypotension is a medical term used to describe low blood pressure. A person with low blood pressure (hypotension) may be subject to dizziness or even occasional fainting spells at high altitudes. Every little exertion may upset the blood circulation or the normal heart activity. In 90 per cent of all cases the symptoms appear as a result of insufficiency of the gonads. In a woman, the ovaries do not function correctly and in a man it is the male sex glands that are out of order. Blood pressure can return to normal when stimulation of glandular activity is given. I am not suggesting here powerful synthetic hormone preparations but natural remedies.

One renowned remedy for low blood pressure is hyssop, a plant that has been known and used since biblical times. Bee pollen too can help increase a low blood pressure due to its stimulating effects on the sex glands. In fact, it is suggested by many leading naturopaths that bee pollen is so effective at raising blood pressure that people with hypertension should never take it as to do so may cause a stoke.

Raw carrot juice is another natural remedy for increasing blood pressure. If carrots are eaten raw or in a salad they will have no effect on the blood pressure it is only the pure juice that is curative. This also applies to beetroot juice.

RECOMMENDATIONS FOR HYPOTENSION

DIET	Small frequent meals, containing all of the major food groups, carbohydrates, essential fatty acids and low fat protein.
INCREASE	Carrot and Beetroot juice. Good sources of complex carbohydrate. Oily fish – sardines salmon, herring, tuna and mackerel.
DECREASE	Everything refined – especially white bread and flour, confectionery, and alcohol.
SUPERFOODS	Medicinal mushrooms, Bee Pollen, Rotate Spirulina, Chlorella and blue-green algae. Barley Grass, and bio-yoghurt
SUPPLEMENTS	Phytoestrogens, Calcium and Magnesium.
HERBALS	Hyssop.
LIFESTYLE CHANGES	Ensure there is adequate protein in the diet at every meal. Take a bath with 4 drops of Geranium essential oil, which is a natural 'hormone balancer'.

OBESITY

Obesity is the medical term used for people who have excess weight above a body mass index of 25. Excess body weight is implicated as a risk factor for many different diseases including heart disease and diabetes, two of the major killers of modern civilisation. Usually caused by eating too much refined carbohydrates and saturated fats in conjunction with exercising too little. However, there are, of course, other causes of obesity. Hormone imbalances play a large role particularly that of the thyroid, but also the adrenals, pancreas and pituitary can play their part. The origins of obesity often lie in early childhood. Statistically, children who are overweight by the age of two turn into fat adults more frequently than their lean friends. Hereditary too, plays its part.

Obesity is on the increase and is a huge subject in its own right. Eating less and exercising more is not always the answer for these unfortunate people. Many clinically obese clients need psychological help so do not give any specific recommendations in this area unless you are qualified and confident to do so. You can however refer them to a specialist in that area.

Societies in which very little fat is eaten have virtually no obesity. Reducing fat, and in particular saturated fat from the diet has to be the most important component of weight loss. Foods with a high proportion of calories from fat should be eliminated or limited in the diet, these include red meat, poultry skins, dark poultry meat, fried foods, butter, margarine, cheese, whole milk, junk foods and most processed foods.

Many people who are diagnosed as obese, do not have eating disorders as such, but many experience *disordered eating*. The first stage of any serious weight-reducing regime is to regulate the eating pattern. Depending upon the client's lifestyle and commitments, he or she would list up to five times in a 24-hour period times which would become regular eating times. Whether hungry or not, the client would eat at these times, which would in time become a habit, resulting in a regular pattern of eating. After an initial period of a couple of weeks of regulating the eating pattern of *when to eat*, then a further address would be made as to what to eat. Many obese and overweight clients know exactly what to eat, they have probably bought every slimming magazine ever written. They need help in breaking old habits permanently, and regulating eating times, has proved an excellent way to begin this process.

Many low calorie diets are also low in nutrients therefore a daily multivitamin is always recommended. Chromium is usually added to the supplement recommendations as it plays an essential role in the metabolism of carbohydrates and in the action of insulin. Chromium in a form called chromium picolinate, has been studied for its potential role in altering body composition and preliminary research in animals and humans[186] [187] suggested that supplementation with chromium picolinate promoted loss of body fat and an increase in muscle mass.

5–Hydroxytryptophan (5–HTP), the precursor to the neurotransmitter serotonin, has been shown in two short-term controlled studies to reduce appetite and to promote weight loss.[188] In one of these studies, a twelve-week double blind trial, overweight women who took 600–900 mg of 5–HTP per day lost significantly more weight than did women who received the placebo.

The herb guarana contains guaranine (which is nearly identical to caffeine) and the closely related alkaloids thebromine and theophylline; these compounds may curb appetite and increase weight loss. Caffeine's effects (and hence those of guaranine) are well known and include stimulating the central nervous system increasing metabolic rate, and producing a mild diuretic effect.[189] Because of concern of potential adverse effects, many nutritional therapists do not advocate using guarana or caffeine-like substances to reduce weight.

Another herb, *Ephedra sinica*, commonly known as ma huang, is also a central nervous system stimulant. Double blind studies have shown that ephedra, particularly when combined with caffeine, promotes weight loss. Again, because of possible adverse effects, especially when combined with caffeine, ma huang is not usually recommended as an aid to weight loss.

The superfood spirulina has been the subject of one double blind study of sixteen overweight individuals who ingested 2.8 grams of spirulina three times per day for four weeks. The results showed a small but statistically significant weight loss.[190]

Many clients with weight problems know that reducing fat in their diet should result in a weight loss. Unfortunately, many of these clients are eating 99per cent fat free foods (that are usually high in salt and hidden sugars) or try to eliminate fat altogether in their diets. It is these clients that need educating in the importance of the right kind of fat in the diet. The essential fatty acids that should make up 10 per cent of daily calorie intake are also anti-inflammatory and health promoting.

Many clients lose weight on weight reducing diets only to gain it again when they resume their 'normal diet'. Encouragement and advice should be given to overweight and obese clients that the weight reducing diet will become a lifelong lifestyle change and should in time become their 'normal diet'.

You can of course greatly assist overweight clients by encouraging them to eat more natural foods, fish and poultry, fruit and vegetables, unpolluted water and partake of gentle regular exercise. You should advocate the benefits of nutritious food against the immense health problems associated with fast-food, adulterated and denatured food and to discourage the overfed but undernourished population we are becoming.

RECOMMENDATIONS FOR OBESITY

DIET	A high fiber, low saturated fat diet.
INCREASE	Fruit, vegetables, oily fish – sardines salmon, herring, tuna and mackerel. Water
DECREASE	Dieter's foods, red meat, hard cheese, all ready-made meals, alcohol, and all refined foods and alcohol.
SUPERFOODS	Algae, especially spirulina. Super Sprouts, Alfalfa, Bee Pollen and Yoghurt
SUPPLEMENTS	Flaxseed fiber. A good multivitamin and mineral containing 50mg of the B vitamins. Chromium.
HERBALS	Ginger, Ginkgo Biloba, Rhodiola
LIFESTYLE CHANGES	Movement – regular gentle daily walking.

VARICOSE VEINS

Disturbances in the venous system are much more frequent than in the arterial system and women especially suffer from stagnation of blood in the veins. The valves of the veins, whose function it is to prevent back-flow, cease to work efficiently and stagnation of blood occurs. The body has an amazing ability to repair itself, given the right conditions and the veins should, like other organs of the body be regenerated rather than removed. The first course of action for varicosed veins is sensible clothing and sensible shoes – with a maximum height of $1\frac{1}{2}$ inches. Clothes should be well fitting and not excessively tight, especially lingerie, as this can constrict circulation. Avoid standing for long periods of time, especially on stone or concrete. If this is unavoidable because of working commitments then good quality insoles should be fitted inside shoes and replaced regularly. A diet rich in vitamins and fresh fruit is, as always, highly recommended. Lastly circulation must be stimulated by regular exercise, thus providing sufficient oxygen for maximum function.

May people who have varicose veins also suffer from constipation and if this is the case then the first course of action is to establish proper bowel elimination.

Although witch hazel is known primarily for combating hemorrhoids it may also be used for varicose veins.[244] Application of witch hazel ointment three or more times per day for two or more weeks should show improvement.

Horse chestnut can be used both internally and as an external application for disordered venous circulation, including varicose veins. Preliminary studies in humans have showed that 300mg three times per day of a standardized extract of horse chestnut can produce some benefit on one aspect of varicose veins.[245]

General care of the legs is of paramount importance. Do not consider putting your feet up as a luxury – look at it as a necessity. Carefully empty the veins by careful stroking and gentle massage in an upward direction. In the evening before going to bed is a good time and using a natural oil, like sweet almond, avocado or St John's Wort, that all have high nutritive values in their own right, will be even more beneficial. Patience and perseverance are needed when treating varicose veins the natural way. It took a long time for them to become varicose in the first place and the harm cannot be reversed overnight.

RECOMMENDATIONS FOR VARICOSE VEINS

DIET	A whole food approach to food where quality is more important than quantity. Plenty of fruits, vegetables, nuts and seeds with low-fat protein and adequate essential fatty acids.
INCREASE	Oily fish – sardines salmon, herring, tuna and mackerel. Plenty of fresh fruit and vegetables – blended in a juicer as well as whole. and low fat protein foods.
DECREASE	Everything refined – especially white bread and flour, confectionery, and alcohol
SUPERFOODS	Alfalfa, Barley Grass, Spirulina
SUPPLEMENTS	Multivitamin and mineral with additional 1g vitamin C daily GLA in Evening Primrose Oil.
HERBALS	Witch hazel and horse chestnut both as an ointment
LIFESTYLE CHANGES	Avoid leg crossing. Keeping legs elevated relieves pain. Avoid sitting or standing for prolonged periods of time and walk regularly.

GENERAL RECOMMENDATIONS FOR
THE CARDOVASCUAR SYSTEM

DIET **FOODS TO SUPPORT**	Oily fish – sardines salmon, herring, tuna and mackerel to be eaten at least three times per week. Garlic, fruits and green leafy vegetables such as kale and broccoli. Olive oil for cooking.
FOODS TO AVOID	Refined foods – those high in white flour and sugar. All foods high in saturated fat such as fatty bacon, fat within meat and 'hidden' fats in biscuits and confectionery. High sodium foods and all alcohol.
SUPERFOODS	Barley Grass, Algae especially spirulina, Super Sprouts, Alfalfa, Bee Pollen and Yoghurt.
SUPPLEMENTS	B-Complex — commonly known as the 'heart healers'. Magnesium Flaxseed Fibre. Branched chain amino acids Co-Q-10, and vitamins E and C.
HERBAL REMEDIES	Garlic Ginkgo Biloba Siberian Ginseng.
LIFESTYLE CHANGES	Regular aerobic exercise – is the most beneficial change you can make to support and strengthen the cardiovascular system. Always check with GP before embarking on any exercise programme.

THE DIGESTIVE SYSTEM

What is the digestive system?

The digestive system is the system of the body that prepares the food we eat ready for absorption by the villi of the small intestine into the body for use by all cells.

Main function

To make food physically small enough and chemically simple enough to be absorbed into the body by the villi and lacteals of the small intestine or to be eliminated out of the body. The terms used for these activities are ingestion, digestion, absorption and defecation.

What does the digestive system actually do?

The digestive system is a complex tube running from the mouth to the anus. It is the only body system that has contact with the outside world from the openings at the mouth and anus.

Everything we put into our mouths has to be chemically changed into a substance that can be absorbed by the small intestine before being transported to the liver.

Digestion starts when we see, smell or just think of food. These senses trigger the brain to start to produce enzymes ready for breaking down food. Thus our mouths start to 'water'. This water is actually saliva in which is found salivary amylase – the enzyme that begins carbohydrate breakdown.

Enzymes are proteins that change one substance into another and there are three types of digestive enzymes. These are amylase that break down carbohydrates, protease that break down proteins and lipase that break down fats. There are many different enzymes within each particular group of enzymes.

When we eat carbohydrates (bread, pasta, fruit, peas, beans, lentils, vegetables) the process of breaking down these foods into substances that we can actually absorb begins in the mouth by the action of salivary amylase. It is of vital important therefore that we allow the food to stay in our mouths long enough for this chemical breakdown to begin and for this enzyme to begin its work.

Thus chemical breakdown begins in the mouth. At the same time mechanical breakdown begins with breaking down the food into smaller pieces by our teeth and tongue. The smaller the food can become in the mouth, the easier it is for the stomach and the remainder of the digestive system to do their job properly.

Once the food has been chewed well, it forms into a ball at the back of the mouth called a bolus, which is then swallowed. It then travels down the oesophagus, through a spincter at the bottom of the oesophagus and directly into the stomach. Liquids take seconds to arrive in the stomach and well-chewed food takes several seconds and reaches the stomach by peristalsis. Peristalsis is an automatic action stimulated by the presence of food and occurs in all sections of the alimentary canal – from the oesophagus through to the large intestine.

Protein digestion does not start until it reaches the stomach, but it is still important to chew protein foods into small pieces. By chewing protein foods (meat, cheese, eggs, fish, and nuts) thoroughly, you are assisting the function of the stomach when the proteins arrive there.

There is a lipase that is produced in the mouth for fat breakdown, but the production is so small that we say that all fat breakdown begins in the duodenum. But as with the carbohydrates and proteins, chewing is of vital importance to assist proper digestion and absorption later.

Unfortunately, this very simple, primitive action of putting food into our mouths and chewing thoroughly and slowly before swallowing is being lost resulting in thousands of people suffering major digestive problems because of not doing this simple act. The consequences of not chewing your food thoroughly are many and varied and may include indigestion, heartburn, bloating, malabsorption, irritable bowel syndrome and constipation to name but a few.

DIGESTIVE SYSTEM RULE NO. 1
Chew Your Food Thoroughly — Always

The main function of the stomach is one of breaking down protein foods into smaller chains, which will finally become amino acids, which can then be absorbed into our bodies. By chewing our food well, the protein that arrives in the stomach should be in quite small pieces. The stomach produces hydrochloric acid, the main function of which is to straighten out the long curly protein chains into smaller molecules. The stomach also produces an enzyme called pepsinogen. This is an inactive enzyme, or else it would start digesting the stomach itself, but when protein food enters the stomach the pepsinogen mixes with the hydrochloric acid and becomes an active enzyme called pepsin. This enzyme can then begin its work and start to break down proteins into di-peptides — smaller chains of proteins.

To put larger pieces of unchewed food, protein in particular, into the stomach is putting an immense strain on this organ and making the function of the pepsin much harder. The food has to stay in the stomach longer making you feel uncomfortable. The carbohydrate eaten with the same meal will also be sitting in the stomach. The salivary amylase works for a little while in the acidic environment of the stomach but then ceases.

Protein breakdown is therefore dependent on hydrochloric acid and pepsinogen mixing together to make pepsin. But what happens if there is not enough hydrochloric acid? Without adequate amounts of hydrochloric acid it is impossible for the protein to be broken-down. A low level of hydrochloric acid is known as hypochloridia and an absence of hydrocloric acid is known as achlorhydria.

Stress plays an important part in the whole digestive process as stress may reduce the production of hydrochloric acid. The symptoms of having too much or too little hydrochloric acid are very similar and it is therefore very difficult to decide if you are producing too much or too little, other than having a clinical test. Many people are diagnosed with producing too much acid and are given antacids to combat the problem. However, if the diagnosis was incorrect and the person was not producing sufficient acid then the problems will be made worse by taking the antacids.

Hydrochloric acid secretion in the stomach in an important part of the digestive process, and interference with this process can be a potential source of malnutrition. Hydrochloric acid is essential for the absorption of several trace minerals most notably calcium and iron.

The problems that start at the beginning of the digestive tract can manifest themselves to more complicated problems further down the tract.

The food eventually passes from the stomach to the duodenum, the first part of the small intestine. Here the environment changes from the acid environment of the stomach to an alkaline environment. Pancreatic enzymes produced by the pancreas achieve this. The pancreas has two functions, one as an endocrine gland and one as an exocrine gland. It produces all three main digestive enzymes — pancreatic protease, amylase and lipase and these enzymes pass directly into the duodenum. At the same time, bile from the bile duct of the liver also enters the duodenum helping to create an alkaline environment.

It is here that the fats from our food begin to be broken down. Bile and pancreatic lipase emulsifies the fat, breaking it down into molecules small enough to be absorbed through the lacteals of the villi. Fats are broken down into glycerol and fatty acids before absorption.

Eventually the food will have been broken down into units physically small enough and chemically simple enough for absorption. Absorption takes place through the villi of the small intestine, which are designed in millions of tiny folds for greater surface absorption area. The carbohydrates and proteins go straight into the bloodstream to the liver and the fats are absorbed through the lacteals and into the lymphatic system.

What is not or cannot be absorbed travels into the large colon via the ileocecal valve. Indigestible fibre makes up most of this bulk which is needed to help carry away unwanted materials of digestion and toxins.

The large colon has four main functions. The absorption of most of the water from the faeces in order to conserve water in the body and form faeces; storage of the faeces, the production of mucous to lubricate the passage of the faeces and the expulsion of the faeces out of the body.

Dietary influences affecting the digestive system

Digestive disorders are on the increase and millions of people are suffering in silence. This is a worrying trend but there is tremendous help available by way of small but permanent lifestyle changes; changes in basic dietary habits and by regularly supplementing and supporting the system with natural products.

The most important dietary influences affecting the digestive system are fiber and water. The fiber in our diets can be described as an 'intestinal broom' as it sweeps the system clean.

The recommended daily intake of water is at least one litre a day and many people struggle to meet this quantity. Many people regard water as merely an uninteresting liquid. However, natural water can provide significant quantities of minerals and spring water in particular is a good source. Water that has been artificially carbonated on the other hand can actually rob our bodies of minerals. Tap water should be avoided as in many areas tap water contains significant levels of nitrates, lead and aluminium. Using a filter only addresses half the problem, as although the nitrates may be removed, so too are the essential minerals. It is imperative therefore that we obtain our minerals from either the foods that we eat or from a dietary supplement.

Many symptoms associated with digestive disorders can signal more serious conditions. A visit to a nutritional therapist or the client's GP for a check-up, should always be recommended.

COLONIC IRRIGATION

Colonic irrigation is a thorough cleaning of the colon, almost like a glorified enema, which is administered by an operator trained and accustomed to this work. The treatment lasts approximately 45 minutes to one hour and during that time water is inserted into the colon through the rectum, at the rate of several ounces at a time, then expelled, before the process is repeated. The therapist can see what has been removed from the colon by a 'glass viewing tube'. By seeing the colour, texture, the size and amount of air bubbles, undigested food and consistency of the fecal matter, many digestive disorders can be ascertained. It is a perfectly safe and painless treatment and can be a valuable diagnostic tool.

COMMON DISORDERS
CELIAC DISEASE

Celiac disease is a hypersensitivity to gluten, which is a protein, found in wheat, rye, barley and oats. Although gluten sensitivity is not a food allergy, individuals with celiac disease avoid foods containing wheat, rye, barley, and oats in the same way those with food allergies avoid the foods to which they are allergic. Celiac disease can also be described as a chronic malabsorption syndrome due to gluten intolerance.

There are many symptoms to celiac disease, the main ones being failure to thrive, weight loss, loss of appetite, vomiting in some cases, diarrhoea, stools that are bulky, pale, frothy and/or foul-smelling; dermatitis, abdominal distention and pain, weakness, and anemia.

For persons with celiac disease the toxic part of the gluten molecule is the prolamin portion being gliadin in wheat, secalin in rye, horedin in barley, and evedin in oats. The gluten found in corn and rice does not contain this toxic portion.

In celiac disease, gluten ingestion results in damage and destruction of the villi. You can visualise the damage by thinking of a shag carpet changing into linoleum. The flattened surface of the small intestine reduces its capacity to digest and absorb nutrients. It changes the lining of the upper part of the intestine, making it less able to absorb nutrients from food. It affects approximately 1 in 1,000 people and is being increasingly recognised. There is no known cure. A gluten-free diet is the only treatment and there must be lifelong adherence to this diet.

RECOMMENDATIONS FOR CELIAC DISEASE

DIET	Strictly no wheat, rye, barley, millet and oats.
INCREASE	Brown rice, millet and corn, brown rice cakes, corn tortillas.
DECREASE	Everything refined – especially white bread and flour, confectionery, and alcohol
SUPERFOODS	Alfalfa, Medicinal Mushrooms, Blue-Green Algae.
SUPPLEMENTS	Multivitamin/mineral liquid formula for better absorption.
HERBALS	Quercetin, Slippery Elm tea.
LIFESTYLE CHANGES	Read labels rigorously.

CONSTIPATION

This is a common problem but a serious one. Constipation is not to do with regularity but more to do with the consistency of the stool. If the bowels move once or twice a day and the stools are hard and difficult to pass, the person is constipated – no matter how regular they are. Constipation results when food moves too slowly through the gastrointestinal tract (GI). The longer the stool is in the body the more concentrated it will become and the more difficult to pass.

A useful index is the time it takes food to pass through the body. In diets of unrefined cereals, fruits and plenty of raw vegetables the transit time is usually 12 hours or so. Fecal matter is bulkier, less dense and easier to pass along the digestive tract. The amount of time food waste is spent inside the body is therefore also decreased. A tablespoon of linseeds taken with breakfast cereal can make passage of stools easier.

If our digestive systems are working efficiently, then every time we eat something, we should go to the toilet soon after. When we see, smell or taste food, then the whole of the digestive system should start working from the oesophagus to the anus. As food enters the oesophagus from the mouth then the entire 'tube' should go into action, by way of peristaltic muscular actions. Unfortunately, due to low fibre diets and convenience foods, this does not always happen and many people often go days before eliminating. Gentle massage around the colon moving in a clockwise direction may help loosen the compacted matter inside the colon. Again, advice may be to see a nutritional therapist, as simply eating more fibre may not be the answer. Less than three bowel actions a week is considered a problem or if a person has to strain to endure a movement. Any change in bowel habit, which occurs for no obvious reason, in people aged around 40 or over should visit their GP, as it could be the sign of a more serious problem.

Many nutritional therapists recommend taking 7.5grams of psyllium seeds or 5 grams psyllium husks, mixed with water or juice, once or twice a day. Some therapists use a combination of senna (18%) and psyllium (82%) for the treatment of chronic constipation. This has been shown to work for people in nursing homes.[35]

One colonic irrigation treatment may be of benefit in cases of chronic constipation. In constipation, peristalsis is inhibited due to the compacted feces, but after a colonic treatment, when much the compacted fecal matter has been eased and removed from the colon, then peristalsis action can be restored.

RECOMMENDATIONS FOR CONSTIPATION

DIET	A diet high in insoluble fiber – vegetables, beans, brown rice, whole wheat, rye, and other whole grains.
INCREASE	Water intake. Brown bread and brown rice
DECREASE	White bread, white rice and alcohol.
SUPERFOODS	Alfalfa, Barley Grass, Chlorophyll, Super sprouts.
SUPPLEMENTS	Flaxseed oil, Psyllium Husks.
HERBALS	Ginger, Aloe, Cascara, Senna Don Quai – naturally relaxes the bowels to speed healing
LIFESTYLE CHANGES	Exercise may increase the muscular contractions of the intestine. Investigate colonic irrigation in your area.

Clients are advised to see their doctor if they have the following symptoms:-

Any change in bowel habit that lasts more than a couple of days

Blood or black matter in the stools

Pain in the abdomen that may or may not be linked to passing stools

Difficulty in controlling bowel movements

CROHN'S DISEASE AND ULCERATIVE COLITIS

Ulcerative Colitis and Crohn's Disease (collectively called Inflammatory Bowel Disease or IBD) are chronic illnesses for which there is at present no known causes or cures.

Both sexes can suffer equally and IBD can strike at any age from the very young child to an older person. There is no known cause for the onset of the symptoms, which will include, pain, diarrhoea, fever, loss of appetite, weight loss, abdominal fullness, incontinence, joint pain, and foul smelling and/or bloody stools.

Incidence of Crohn's disease is rising particularly among young people. It is now thought that IBD affect over 120,000 people in the UK with 8,000 new cases each year. Diagnosis is complicated and other diseases must be first ruled out. Treatment for both conditions involves a healthy balanced diet, particularly important after a severe attack to replace lost nutrients. Crohn's disease is limited to the small intestine in 90 per cent of cases.

The cause of Crohn's disease is said to be unknown, but overeating, chemical poisoning, or bacterial invasion all seem to be possible factors or etiologic agents.[30] Substantially greater numbers of people with the disease give a history of using more refined sugar, less dietary fiber, and considerably less raw fruit and vegetables than the controls. This kind of diet favours the development of Crohn's disease.[31][32][33] Some investigators point out that sugary foods tend to contain more chemical additives such as dyes, flavours, and stabilisers. These investigators also suggest that a high sugar intake itself may influence the intestinal bacteria flora to produce compounds toxic to the intestinal lining.[34]

Exercise is important and should include daily walking whenever possible.

Avoid any gas-forming foods such as cabbage, corn, certain greens, pickles and relishes of all kinds, skins of apples, potatoes, and legumes. It is well to try an elimination diet to determine if one is sensitive to any group of the most common foods causing sensitivity. Milk and all dairy products including whey products, sodium lactate, sodium casenate and all other milk residues should also be avoided, as an allergy to dairy produce is very common with Crohn's disease. Avoidance of all spices, food additives, dyes, preservatives and stimulants such as coffee, tea, cola, and alcohol should all be avoided.

A small percentage of patients suffer from uveitis, a painful inflammation of the eye. This complication usually improves when the IBD is brought under control. A physician should always evaluate any inflammation of the eye.

RECOMMENDATIONS FOR CROHN'S DISEASE & ULCERATIVE COLITIS

DIET	A bland, low-fat diet should be instituted
INCREASE	Liberal quantities of complex carbohydrates – fruits (without the skins), vegetables and whole grains.
DECREASE	Milk and cheese should be avoided, and all refined foods. Ideally there should be no saturated fats, no fried foods, no sugar and no extremely hot or cold foods.
SUPERFOODS	Alfalfa, Bee Pollen, Spirulina, Chlorella and Blue-Green Algae – rotate one month on each.
SUPPLEMENTS	A complex of Omega 3 and 6 fatty acids and Probiotics
HERBALS	Ginger – relieves gas and settles stomach. Quercetin
LIFESTYLE CHANGES	All foods should be chewed well, or mashed with a fork, or pureed in a blender. Two meals a day are preferable to three as proper digestion and assimilation are more vital. Consider allergy testing to identify any substances you may be sensitive to.

DIARRHOEA

Any attack of frequent watery stools is called diarrhoea, and many different conditions can cause it. Diarrhoea is often a symptom of gastro-intestinal distress caused by bacteria. In cases like this, probiotics may normalise bowel function by neutralising infectious microorganisms.

Allergies and food sensitivities are common triggers for diarrhoea.[36] For example some infants suffer diarrhoea when fed a cow's milk-based formula but improve when switched to soy-based formula.[37]

People with chronic diarrhoea not attributable to other causes should discuss the possibility of food sensitivity with a nutritional therapist who specialises in allergies.

Drinking lots of coffee causes diarrhoea in some people.[38] People with chronic diarrhoea who drink coffee should avoid all coffee for a few days to evaluate whether coffee is the cause.

The malabsorption problems that develop during diarrhoea can lead to deficiencies of vitamins and minerals.[39] For this reason it makes sense for people with diarrhoea to try a multiple vitamin/mineral supplement. Two of the nutrients that may not absorb as a result of diarrhoea are zinc and vitamin A, both needed to fight infections. In third world countries supplementation with zinc and vitamin A has lead to a reduction in or prevention of infections diarrhoea.[40] Whether such supplementation would help people in less deficient population remains unclear.

Some foods contain sugars that absorb slowly such as fructose in fruit juice or sorbitol in diabetic confectionery. Through a process of osmosis, these unabsorbed sugars hold onto water in the intestines, sometimes leading to diarrhoea.[41] By reading labels, people with chronic non-infectious diarrhoea can easily avoid fruit juice, fructose, and sorbitol to see if this eliminates the problem.

People who are lactose intolerant, meaning they lack the enzyme needed to digest milk sugar, often develop diarrhoea after consuming milk or ice cream. People whose lactose intolerance is the cause of diarrhoea will rid themselves of the problem by avoiding milk and ice cream or in many cases by taking lactase, the enzyme needed to digest lactose. Lactase is available in a variety of forms from health food stores.

Large amounts of vitamin C or magnesium found in supplements can also cause diarrhoea although the amount varies considerably from person to person. Unlike infectious diarrhoea, other signs of illness do not generally accompany diarrhoea caused by high amounts of vitamin C or magnesium. The same is true when the problem comes from sorbitol or fructose.[42]

Carob is rich in tannins that have an astringent or binding effect on the mucous membranes of the intestinal tract. It is often used for young children and infants with diarrhoea, and a double blind study suggests it is effective. Commonly, 15 grams of carob powder is mixed with applesauce (for flavour) when given to children. Carob can also be used for adult diarrhoea.

Chamomile reduces intestinal cramping and eases the irritation and inflammation associated with diarrhoea, according to test tube studies.[43] Chamomile is typically drunk as tea, but many nutritional therapists recommend dissolving 2–3 grams of powdered chamomile or adding 3–5 ml of a chamomile liquid extract to hot water and drinking it three or more times per day, between meals. Alternatively, two to three teaspoons of the dried flowers can be steeped in a cup of hot water and covered for ten to fifteen minutes before drinking.

Diarrhoea can also be the result from food poisoning, gastroenteritis, anxiety, antibiotic treatment, excess alcohol or Irritable Bowel Syndrome. Other more rare conditions can cause chronic diarrhoea, including some bowel cancers and hormonal changes such as diabetes, so it is important that sufferers seek medical attention if diarrhoea goes on for more than a few days.

RECOMMENDATIONS FOR DIARRHOEA

DIET	A whole food approach to food where quality is more important than quantity. Plenty of fruits, vegetables, nuts and seeds with adequate essential fatty acids, low-fat protein, and plenty of water.
INCREASE	Dietary fiber.
DECREASE	Fruit juice, fructose and sorbitol.
SUPERFOODS	Alfalfa, Medicinal mushrooms, Barley Grass, Yoghurt, Super sprouts.
SUPPLEMENTS	Multivitamin/mineral to protect against deficiencies Folic acid, Brewer's Yeast, Probiotics. Lactase for lactose intolerant people
HERBALS	Carob, Chamomile
LIFESTYLE CHANGES	Control stress levels by taking up yoga. Meditation and visualisation techniques may also help.

DIVERTICULITIS

Diverticula are saclike pouches on the wall of the large colon in places where the muscularis has become weak. The development of diverticula is called diverticulosis. Many people who develop this condition are asymptomatic and experience no complications. About 15 percent of people with diverticulosis will eventually develop an inflammation within diverticula, a condition then known as diverticulitis. Research indicates that diverticula form because of lack of sufficient bulk in the colon. The powerful contractions, working against insufficient bulk, create a high pressure that it causes the colonic walls to bulge.[113]

Symptoms are usually pain above the right hip area of the abdomen, nausea, vomiting and abdominal distention, constipation and/or diarrhoea. Most common causes are fibre deficiency, refined diet, white bread, and white rice, nutritional deficiency in general and muscular weakness in intestinal walls. Constipation and obesity are considerations, as are poor bowel habits. An allergy, especially to dairy products, is also indicated in some people.

Recommendations should only be given after referral from the client's GP. In the meantime, a liquid multivitamin would be recommended. It is also important to regulate eating times – little and often with quality rather than quantity being of paramount importance. The following recommendations are for clients with established diverticulitis, that is, once the condition is under control, as the initial treatment could be a *low fiber* diet followed by introductions to higher fiber foods.

RECOMMENDATIONS FOR DIVERTICULITIS

DIET	A whole food approach to food where quality is more important than quantity. Plenty of fruits, vegetables, nuts and seeds with adequate essential fatty acids, low-fat protein, and plenty of water.
INCREASE	Bran flakes (if no wheat sensitivity). Oily fish – sardines salmon, herring, tuna and mackerel. Dietary fiber.
DECREASE	Refined foods including white bread and rice.
SUPERFOODS	Alfalfa, Medicinal mushrooms, Chlorophyll, bio-yoghurt.
SUPPLEMENTS	A liquid multivitamin and mineral Vitamins E and C. Probiotics – can be bought powdered to mix up into a drink.
HERBALS	Garlic, preferably raw in salads. Slippery elm tea and Marshmallow.
LIFESTYLE CHANGES	The daily consumption of six to eight large glasses of water *every day*, is a very useful aid to proper bowel function and the most important lifestyle change you can make.

DYSBIOSIS

Dysbiosis describes the state of health of the internal human gastrointestinal system. Everything that enters the mouth ultimately undergoes various forms of digestion. Any imbalance within the human gastrointestinal system will disturb not only digestion but predisposes people to nutritional deficiencies and numerous related health problems.

This occurs particularly when pathogenic microorganisms take up residence in the spaces located between the villi of the small intestine. Each species of microorganism produces potentially harmful digestive by-products and toxic chemical compounds that can be absorbed into the blood stream, causing a predisposition to health problems, which are often undiagnosed or misdiagnosed. Many people who have food allergies, dietary irregularities and nutritional imbalances have, unknown to them, internal gastrointestinal putrefactive dysbiosis producing generations of toxic chemicals. These chemicals not only alter digestion but also allow those toxic chemicals to enter the blood stream and cause systemic health problems.

As assessment of the gut wall can be undertaken at many nutritional laboratories throughout the country to determine the permeability of the gut. The test employs the use of an oral challenge containing a mixed molecular carbohydrate solution of various sized molecules. Depending upon the size of molecules collected in a urine sample after the challenge, the laboratory is able to assess the degree of gastro-intestinal permeability in the sufferer.

Treatment is quite straightforward. The first stage is to remove the cause, followed by improving the gut function before healing the gut wall.

Removing the cause may mean making significant changes to lifestyle, including the avoidance of food allergens and over-use of caffeine, alcohol and other anti-nutrients. Improving the gut function is accomplished by improving the general diet and finally healing the gut is usually done with various supplements.

L-Glutamine is one such supplement. It is the most abundant amino acid in plasma and is used as a major fuel source in rapidly replicating tissues such as the intestinal lining. L-Glutamine is now considered a semi-essential amino acid in human nutrition. This supplement improves gut barrier function and therefore is an invaluable component in the leaky gut syndrome treatment programme. L-Glutamine supplements repair damage to the intestines from diseases like colitis, irritable bowel syndrome, celiac disease, Crohn's disease and any condition affecting digestion.

A study from the *British Journal of Surgery* showed that L-Glutamine improves conditions similar to inflammatory bowel disease in laboratory animals by significantly decreasing the permeability of the intestinal lining

HEALTH PROBLEMS RELATED TO DYSBIOSIS

Arthritis	Diabetes	Indigestion	Pimples
Acne	Diarrhoea	Impotence	Psoriasis
Alcoholism	Drug Addiction	Infections	Sinusitis
Allergies	Dysmennorrhea	IBS	Skin rashes
Anemia	Earaches	Cystitis	Septicemia
Anorexia	Eczema	Insomnia	Weakness
Asthma	Endometriosis	Joint Pains	Incontinence
ADS*	Epilepsy	Lactose Intolerance	Uterine cysts
Anxiety	Fibrocitis	Loss of Hair	Uterine Fibroids
Back problems	Fibromyalgia	Loss of Libido	Vaginitis
Bulimia	Gastritis	Loss of Memory	Lupus
Candidiasis	Headaches	Meningitis	Menstrual problems
Cancer	Hypoglycemia	Mood swings	Muscle aches
Constipation	Hormone problems	Nervousness	Obesity
Colitis	Hyperactivity	Osteoporosis	Pains

*Attention Deficit Syndrome

RECOMMENDATIONS FOR DYSBIOSIS

DIET	A whole food approach to food where quality is more important than quantity. Plenty of fruits, vegetables, nuts and seeds with adequate essential fatty acids, low-fat protein, and plenty of water.
INCREASE	Raw fruits and vegetables.
DECREASE	All refined 'denatured' foods, salt, sugar, coffee, tea, chocolate, confectionery and alcohol.
SUPERFOODS	Rotate Spirulina, Chlorella and Blue-Green Algae. Yoghurt, Alfalfa, Medicinal mushrooms, Barley Grass.
SUPPLEMENTS	Probiotics — taken in powder form mixed up into a drink. L-Glutamine — used for cell growth and repair.
HERBALS	Garlic, Milk Thistle, Dandelion Coffee and tincture
LIFESTYLE CHANGES	Avoid alcohol, and all stimulants. Consider a 'gut permeability' test to establish the permeability of your gut wall.

FLATULENCE

Flatulence is abnormal amounts of gas passing upwards or downwards with or without intestinal discomfort. The symptoms are excess gas, abdominal distention and discomfort. Flatulence is usually caused by improper diet by way of excess acidity, poor food combinations, beans, hurried meals, frequent meals, allergies or too much liquid drank with meals. It may also be caused by digestive enzyme deficiency, inadequate mastication, poor elimination, or abnormal intestinal flora/yeast overgrowth.

Flatulence is a sign that the digestive system is not working efficiently. Food will not have been completely digested, or digested inadequately by the time it gets to the large colon, so this organ is unable to do its job properly. Digestive enzymes are essential in the digestive process to break down complex proteins, fats, and carbohydrates into small molecules for proper absorption. The result of foods that are too complex passing through the gastro-intestinal tract and into the large intestine, is fermentation, gas and abdominal pain.

Diet is therefore of the utmost importance in all cases of flatulence. Beans are a common problem for many people. They contain oligosaccharides, which have digestive enzyme-resistant chemical bonds between the sugar molecules causing food to be incompletely broken down and passed into the small intestine where fermentation and gas may result. By soaking the beans overnight should overcome this problem.

ACID/ALKALINE BALANCE

Mention is made throughout this book of acid/alkaline balance. Ideally, our diets should make up 80 per cent alkaline forming foods and 20 per cent acid forming foods. However this can be difficult for many people. Initially aim for a 50/50 ratio with your ultimate aim to reach an 80/20 alkaline/acid ratio. Your health will improve the more alkaline forming foods you eat.

Alkaline *forming* foods are not the same as alkaline foods measuring the pH value of the food with litmus paper. The alkaline forming foods may be acid before digestion such as citrus fruits, but after digesting and metabolising they leave an alkaline ash. Alkaline forming foods are emphasised in raw fruit (including grapefruit, lemon and orange) and vegetables, whole grains, almonds, avocados, and some milk products especially yoghurt.

High acid forming diets are negative to good health and induce calcium loss. Most protein foods (bacon, beef, chicken, liver, eggs) are acid forming as well as some grains, brazil nuts, walnuts, hard cheese, olives and shellfish. Alcohol also induces excess acid and has been shown to create a negative calcium balance.

Tea, coffee, sugar, butter and margarine are classed as neutral foods in this connection.

RECOMMENDATIONS FOR FLATULENCE

DIET	A whole food approach to food where quality is more important than quantity. Plenty of fruits, vegetables, nuts and seeds with adequate essential fatty acids, low-fat protein, and plenty of water. Beans soaked overnight then cooked in fresh water usually lose their gas-forming characteristics. Chew foods well
INCREASE	Fruits and vegetables, and sufficient water.
DECREASE	All refined foods. Fried foods, hydrogenated fats, all junk food.
SUPERFOODS	Slippery elm tea, Wild Yam Root tincture
SUPPLEMENTS	None specifically but digestive enzymes help initially. Flaxseed fiber.
HERBALS	None specifically although ginger assists the entire digestive system.
LIFESTYLE CHANGES	Never eat until full and never rush your meals. Chew all foods very well and do not drink liquids, especially milk, while eating. The liquids dilute the digestive juices and hinder proper digestion, often resulting in flatulence

HEARTBURN

Heartburn is described very much as it feels — as a burning pain in the upper chest area over where the heart is — however, it is usually nothing to do with the heart at all. Heartburn is a common way to describe indigestion or 'too much acid'. If it is an excess of hydrochloric acid, the acid may well give a burning feeling. If you have clients with these symptoms advise them to see a nutritional therapist.

Heartburn can however be a symptom of *too little acid.* The symptoms of too much acid and too little acid are very similar and it is difficult to differentiate between the two.

With hypochlorhydria (low stomach acid) it is undigested protein foods causing the trouble. Due to a *lack of* hydrochloric acid in the stomach, the stomach is unable to function as it should by breaking down the long curly protein molecules into smaller chains. The protein food will therefore just sit in the stomach making you feel uncomfortable with the accompanying burning feeling. Many clients only get heartburn after a protein meal.

This may seem a paradox but based on the clinical experience of doctors, supplementing with betain HCl relieves the symptoms of heartburn and improves digestion.[99]

Another cause of heartburn is a condition called hiatus hernia. With this condition a small portion of the stomach gets caught in the sphincter that separates the oesophagus from the stomach. A hiatus hernia usually does not require any specific therapy, but anyone suffering from one with accompanying reflux, should be receiving treatment.

To relieve heartburn some people try antacids, which often provide symptom relief. However, antacids can have their own side effects, since they can interfere with the absorption of some vitamins and minerals. Many antacids also contain aluminium and there has been several conclusive trials indicating that there may be a link between aluminium and Alzheimer's disease. Of course if you take antacids to reduce acidity in the stomach, but in fact you have hypochlorhydria and are producing *insufficient* acid, then by taking the antacids will only make the situation worse.

A potentially beneficial category of herbs for people with indigestion and/or low stomach acid are called bitters. Gentian, dandelion, blessed thistle, yarrow, devil's claw, bitter orange, and centaury are thought to stimulate digestive function by increasing saliva production and promoting both stomach acid and digestive enzyme production.[44] Bitters are taken either by mixing 1–3 ml tincture into water and sipping slowly ten to fifteen minutes before eating, or by taking a tea from the dried herbs, which is also sipped slowly before eating.

RECOMMENDATIONS FOR HEARTBURN

DIET	No specific diet required for heartburn. Ensure that protein foods are chewed well. Stir-fry is a good choice for people suffering with heartburn as the protein is already in smaller pieces, assisting the stomach with its function.
INCREASE	Raw food that contains their own enzymes for better digestion. Brown rice.
DECREASE	Refined foods of all types, and acid forming foods like meat, cheese and milk until the problem has been rectified.
SUPERFOODS	Cabbage. Pineapple contains the enzyme bromelain that assists in the breakdown of protein foods.
SUPPLEMENTS	Betain HCl, or digestive enzymes containing betain HCl. Lactase (for lactose intolerance only). Lecithin. Zinc
HERBALS	Bitters, Goldenseal, Slippery elm tea.
LIFESTYLE CHANGES	Avoid high protein meals. Eat slowly not under stressful conditions, and chew all food well. Smaller meals more frequently are more beneficial than fewer large meals.

DIGESTIVE SYSTEM RULE NO. 2
Never eat under stressful conditions or until you are full.

> **TAKE CARE**
> Peppermint oil, in large amounts, can cause burning and
> gastrointestinal upset in some people. It should be avoided by people
> with chronic heartburn.

HYPOCHLORHYDRIA (Low Stomach Acid)

As explained under 'heartburn', hypochlorhydria is a condition where there is low stomach acid, and the symptoms of too little opposed to too much are very difficult to differentiate. However, low stomach acid is very common, due to the fact that hydrochloric acid is dependent upon zinc, and many people are zinc deficient, due to poor soil conditions and intensive farming. Stress, parasites and B12 deficiency may also be associated with low stomach acid.

Medical researchers since the 1930s have been concerned with the consequences of too little stomach acid. While all the health consequences are still not entirely clear, some have been well documented. Many minerals and vitamins require proper stomach acid to be absorbed optimally. Examples are iron,[45] calcium,[46 47] zinc,[48] and B-complex vitamins,[49] including folic acid[50]. People with achlorhydria (no stomach acid) or hypochlorhydria (low stomach acid) maybe at risk for developing certain mineral deficiencies. Since minerals are important not only for body structure (as in bones and teeth), to activate enzymes (such as superoxide dismutase) and hormones (such as insulin), deficiencies can lead to many health problems.

One of the major tasks of stomach acid is to break proteins down to the point that pancreatic proteolytic enzymes can easily work. If this does not occur, these proteins could be absorbed as more complicated chains. This absorption has been suggested by some researchers to be a major cause of immunological stress and food allergies.[51 52]

In addition, partially digested protein provides a favourable environment for 'unfriendly' bacteria that live in the colon.[53 54] Some of these bacteria produce toxic substances that can be absorbed by the body.

If there is doubt as to too much acid or too little acid, there is clinical tests that can be done very easily. (*see Appendix 1*)

RECOMMENDATIONS FOR HYPOCHLORIDIA (LOW STOMACH ACID)

DIET	No specific diet required for low stomach acid. Ensure that protein foods are chewed well. Stir-fry is a good choice for people suffering with low stomach acid as the protein is already in smaller pieces, assisting the stomach with its function.
INCREASE	Raw food that contains their own enzymes for better digestion.
DECREASE	Refined foods of all types, and acid forming foods like meat, cheese and milk until the problem has been rectified.
SUPERFOODS	Cabbage. Pineapple contains the enzyme bromaline that assists in the breakdown of protein foods.
SUPPLEMENTS	Betain HCl, or digestive enzymes containing betain HCl. Zinc Lactase (for lactose intolerance only).
HERBALS	Bitters, Peppermint, Slippery elm tea.
LIFESTYLE CHANGES	Avoid high protein meals. Eat slowly not under stressful conditions, and chew all food well.

DIGESTIVE SYSTEM RULE NO 3
It takes 20 minutes for your stomach to tell the brain it is full –
Wait before ordering desert. Listen and act to what your body is
telling you

INDIGESTION

Similar to heartburn but the symptoms are not as severe. Eating too quickly and under stressful conditions can cause indigestion. By following Digestive Rule No 2 *never eat under stressful conditions,* and by eating slowly and chewing food very well, indigestion can be avoided.

Artichoke is a mildly bitter plant and healthy food. Extracts of it have been repeatedly shown in double blind research to be beneficial for people with indigestion.[55] Artichoke is particularly useful when the problem is lack of bile production by the liver.[56] Extracts providing 500–1,000mg per day of cynarin, the main active constituent of artichoke, are recommended by many nutritional therapists.

Turmeric, the bright yellow herb we use for colouring rice and other food, has also been used in trials in Thailand. The results from a double blind study showed it relieved indigestion problems.

RECOMMENDATIONS FOR INDIGESTION

DIET	No specific diet required for indigestion. Good well-balanced meals covering all the major food groups.
INCREASE	Raw food that contains their own enzymes for better digestion.
DECREASE	Refined foods of all types, and acid forming foods like meat, cheese and milk until the problem has been rectified.
SUPERFOODS	Cabbage. Pineapple contains the enzyme bromaline that assists in the breakdown of protein foods.
SUPPLEMENTS	Digestive enzymes containing all three types of enzyme. Lactase (for lactose intolerance only)
HERBALS	Bitters, Peppermint, Slippery elm tea.
LIFESTYLE CHANGES	Avoid high protein meals. Eat slowly not under stressful conditions, and chew all food well.

IRRITABLE BOWEL SYNDROME

This is a disease of the entire gastrointestinal tract, and probably the most common gastrointestinal disorder. The main symptoms of IBS are constipation and diarrhoea, and/or uncomfortable bloating. Excessive amounts of mucus may appear in the stools, and other symptoms include flatulence, nausea and loss of appetite. Often how the client actually got IBS can be a mystery. There may be a connection with allergies or food sensitivities with some clients. Anxiety, depression and stress can also be related to IBS. Yeasts and bacteria in the gut emit carbon dioxide and methane gas as natural by products of respiration, and this is often a cause for bloating.

Although increased fiber intake can be helpful in IBS, many sufferers are sensitive to wheat in any form, including wheat bran.[57] [58] [59] Rye, brown rice, oatmeal, and barley are high in hypoallergenic fiber, as are vegetables and psyllium husk.

Some young women with IBS experience worsening symptoms before and during their menstrual periods. Taking evening primrose oil capsules or tables containing 350–400mg of gamma linolenic acid (GLA), the active ingredient, may help such women.[61]

Enteric-coated peppermint oil capsules, providing 0.2ml of peppermint oil, have been shown in some, but not all, studies to be an effective symptomatic treatment for IBS.[62] Many people take one to two capsules three times per day, between meals. The enteric coating protects the peppermint oil while it passes through the acid environment of the stomach. In the intestinal tract, peppermint oil acts as a carminative, eases intestinal cramping, and soothes irritation. Peppermint may also be taken as a tincture in the amount of 2–3ml three times a day.

Chamomile acts as a carminative as well as soothing and toning the digestive tract. Chamomile's essential oils also ease intestinal cramping and irritation.[63] It is often used for those with IBS experiencing alternative bouts of diarrhoea and constipation. Chamomile is typically taken in a tea form by dissolving 2–3 grams of powdered chamomile or by adding 3–5ml of herb extract tincture to hot water, three times per day, between meals. Supplements that combine an assortment of carminative herbs are often useful for IBS. A combination of peppermint leaves, fennel seeds, caraway seeds, and wormwood may be an effective treatment for upper abdominal complaints, including IBS.[64] Some people with IBS benefit from bulk-forming laxatives. Psyllium, mentioned above, helps regulate normal bowel activity and reduces the alternating constipation and diarrhoea suffered by some people with IBS.

RECOMMENDATIONS FOR IBS

DIET	A good well balanced diet covering all food groups but taking care to avoid foods you know liable to disagree.
INCREASE	Brown rice, rye, oatmeal and barley.
DECREASE	White bread and rice, all refined foods. Spicy foods.
SUPERFOODS	Alfalfa, rotate — Spirulina, Chlorella and Blue-Green Algae
SUPPLEMENTS	Probiotics, Evening Primrose or Starflower oil.
HERBALS	Chamomile, Ginger, Peppermint.
LIFESTYLE CHANGES	Identify food intolerances from an experienced practitioner. Practicing stress management skills can be beneficial. Hypnosis for relaxation may also be helpful for those with IBS[60]

MALABSORPTION/UNDERWEIGHT

Malabsorption can be quite difficult to identify and to help. It is often found in people who tend to continually eat, but never seem to put on any weight. Whilst many people like this are in good health, there are many others who have very inefficient digestive systems and are absorbing very little of the food, and therefore nutrients, they are consuming. Digestive enzyme deficiency is often one factor in malabsorption and quite often can be connected to food allergies or sensitivities. This is one condition I immediately investigate when clients come to see me are eating a really good balanced diet, but are quite obviously not at all well in themselves.

Malabsorption syndromes due to allergy or food insensitivity are also very common.

Endocrine imbalances are sometimes responsible for clients not putting on weight and also hypoglycemic and diabetic clients have a particularly difficult time maintaining proper weight.

Zinc deficiency has been known to reduce the appetite and stress and/ or emotionally based weight loss may require psychological help.

Recommend zinc 15mg taken in the evenings and a B-Complex of up to 50mg taken in the mornings.

Gut Permeability Test — this is a urine test that is done in the privacy of your own home and sent directly off to a laboratory for testing. To test, you drink a tasteless solution of various sized molecules and then collect six hours of urine (best done on a Sunday or day off work). A small sample is then collected from the 6-hour collection and sent off to the laboratory, in a specially provided container and packaging.

From the results the laboratory can see how permeable the small intestine is by measuring the size of molecule that has been absorbed. It will show either a very permeable gut, where the client may be experiencing allergy type symptoms, or by contrast, a gut where the villi (small protrusions in the gut where absorption takes place) are atrophied causing some degree of malabsorption. This may lead to gluten intolerance, as it is the gluten from wheat and other grains, that has 'stuck together' the villi of the small intestine. If this is the case then unabsorbed foodstuffs will probably be passing down into the large colon, causing irritation, and over the years either IBS or colitis may result.

Once it has been established by the clinical test how permeable the gut wall is, deciding on a course of action is much easier.

RECOMMENDATIONS FOR
MALABSORPTION/UNDERWEIGHT

DIET	A whole food approach to food where quality is more important than quantity. Plenty of fruits, vegetables, nuts and seeds with adequate essential fatty acids, low-fat protein, and plenty of water.
INCREASE	Adequate and complete proteins are essential.
DECREASE	Everything refined – especially white bread and flour, confectionery, and alcohol.
SUPERFOODS	Alfalfa, Algae, Barley Grass, Medicinal mushrooms, Super sprouts, bio-yoghurt.
SUPPLEMENTS	Digestive Enzymes and probiotics.
HERBALS	Ginger, Quercetin.
LIFESTYLE CHANGES	Rule out food sensitivities or food allergies. Colonic irrigation can be a useful treatment and diagnostic aid to check for undigested foods in the stool.

ULCERS

An ulcer is a craterlike lesion in a membrane and the common symptoms are a burning pain, heartburn, or local tenderness. Ulcers that develop in areas of the gastrointestinal tract exposed to acid gastric juice are called peptic ulcers. Peptic ulcers occasionally develop at the lower end of the oesophagus, but most occur on the lesser curvature of the stomach, where they are called gastric ulcers, or in the first part of the duodenum, where they are called duodenal ulcers which are the most common. Peptic ulcers therefore result when the stomach's digestive juices break the normal defense mechanisms and eat away at the lining of the stomach or duodenum. These ulcers often bleed and may cause sharp burning pain in the area of stomach or just below it. Peptic ulcers should never be treated without proper diagnosis.

About 1 in 10 men and 1 in 15 women have an ulcer at some stage in their life. Too much stomach acid is not always the cause.

Another prime culprit is thought to be the bacteria called *Helicobacter pyori*. People with pectic ulcers due to infection should discuss conventional treatment directed toward eradicating the infection with a medical doctor.

Ulcers can be caused or exacerbated by stress, alcohol smoking and dietary factors. Aspirin and related drugs,[65] alcohol,[66] coffee[67] (including decaf)[68] and tea[69] are known to increase stomach acidity, which can interfere with the healing of an ulcer. Smoking is known to slow ulcer healing.[70.] Whether or not an ulcer is caused by infection, people with peptic ulcer should avoid use of these substances.

Many years ago researchers reported that cabbage juice accelerated healing of peptic ulcers.[71] [72] [73] [74] Drinking up to 5 x 6oz of cabbage juice per day was necessary for symptom relief. Although only preliminary modern research supports this aproach[75] nutritionally oriented doctors and nutritional therapists claim considerable success using this quantity of cabbage juice every day for fourteen days with ulcer symptoms frequently decreasing in only a few days. Carrot juice may be added to improve the flavour. Cabbage juice contains metioninic acid which helps to normalise the mucous membrane in both stomach and duodenum. Drink as much as you can – up to 5 x 6oz glasses daily which can be mixed half-and-half with either carrot juice or celery juice. This is a very soothing drink.

Food allergies have also been linked to peptic ulcers.[76] Exposing the lining of the stomach to foods a person was known to be allergic to has caused bleeding in the stomach.[77] If triggered by *Helicobacter pylori* infection nor helped by other natural approaches, peptic ulcers may respond to avoidance of allergens. Consultation with a nutritional therapist specialising in allergies to ascertain those allergies would be the first course of action.

Garlic,[78] thyme tea and cinnamon tincture have all been reported to have anti-*Helicobacter pylori* activity in test tube studies.[79] Whether these substances would be effective in humans with peptic ulcers caused by this bacterium has yet to be explored in clinical research, but many nutritional therapists use these products with excellent results.

Slippery elm and comfrey teas also come highly recommended. Slippery elm soothes and heals mucous membranes and comfrey contains allantoin, a cell proliferant.

RECOMMENDATIONS FOR ULCERS

DIET	High fiber diet with plenty of fruit and vegetables.
INCREASE	Bananas and unsweetened banana chips, cabbage
DECREASE	Sugar, salt alcohol, hot spices, chocolate, nicotine, tea, coffee, and red meats.
SUPERFOODS	Cabbage especially the juice, Liquorice root
SUPPLEMENTS	Vitamin A, Zinc and Copper in a balanced dose. L-Glutamine.
HERBALS	Garlic, Quercetin, Goldenseal – stops infection, and internal bleeding, eliminates toxins from the stomach.
LIFESTYLE CHANGES	Reduce stress, and never eat under stressful conditions. Identify any allergens and remove these from the diet until the ulcer is repaired. Exchange coffee and tea to strong Chamomile tea, preferably made with a tincture.

GENERAL RECOMMENDATIONS FOR
THE DIGESTIVE SYSTEM

DIET **FOODS TO SUPPORT**	Rice bran, fruits and vegetables, prunes, figs, dates, chicory, artichoke, onion, leek, asparagus, peaches and bananas.
FOODS TO AVOID	All refined foods high in white flour, sugar salt and saturated fat. All spicy foods.
SUPERFOODS	Alfalfa, Spirulina, Cabbage especially the juice, Liquorice root, Manuka Honey and bio-yoghurt.
SUPPLEMENTS	Vitamin C and Folic Acid Probiotics and Prebiotics Digestive enzymes.
HERBAL REMEDIES	Garlic, Quercetin, Goldenseal, Chamomile, Ginger, Peppermint.
LIFESTYLE CHANGES	Make time to sit down at the table to eat. Never eat under stressful conditions and to always eat slowly, chewing your food well.

THE ENDOCRINE SYSTEM

What is the Endocrine system?

The endocrine system is the system of the body that is responsible for releasing chemical messengers, known as hormones, into the bloodstream.

Main function

As one of the main control systems of the body, the other being the nervous system, the endocrine system's main function is that of transmitting messages.

What does the Endocrine system actually do?

The endocrine system sends messages to cells in virtually every part of the body. The endocrine system brings about changes in the metabolic activities of almost all body tissues. The endocrine glands make up the endocrine system. The endocrine glands of the body include the pituitary, thyroid, parathyroids, adrenals, pineal, and thymus gland. In addition there are several organs of the body than contain endocrine tissue but are not exclusively endocrine glands. These include the pancreas, ovaries, testes, kidneys, stomach, small intestine, skin, heart and placenta.

The body contains two kinds of glands: exocrine and endocrine. Exocrine glands secrete their products into ducts, and the ducts carry the secretions into body cavities or to the body's surface. Exocrine glands include sudoriferous (sweat), sebaceous (oil), mucous, and digestive glands. Endocrine glands, on the other hand, secrete their products (hormones) into the extracellular space around the secretory cells, rather than into ducts. The secretion then passes into capillaries to be transported in the blood to target organs.

Dietary influences affecting the endocrine system

The main dietary factor to influence the endocrine system has to be that of synthetic chemicals, many of which mimic the body's hormones, which severely disrupt the system. There are now over 100,000 synthetic chemicals on the international market including 15,000 chlorinated compounds such as PCBs. Some of these are put directly into food; others are added indirectly, in the form of pesticide. Some creep into our food from packaging (especially plastics and cling film) and processing and some we take as medicine. Many of these mimic the role of oestrogen in the body, stimulating the growth of hormone-sensitive tissue such as breast tissue which then increase the risk of hormone-related cancers. These synthetic chemicals that mimic our own hormones confuse and disrupt the endocrine and nervous systems.

ENDOCRINE SYSTEM RULE NO 1
Avoid all synthetic hormones – as they disrupt the Endocrine system

---

COMMON DISORDERS
DIABETES

Diabetes is essentially too much sugar in the blood. There are two types. Type I diabetics must take insulin injections because their pancreas produces virtually no insulin. Type I is also known as insulin dependent or juvenile diabetes.

Type II diabetes accounts for 75 per cent of all cases affecting some one million Britons, and usually develops after the age of 40. Sufferers usually have sufficient insulin but the body cells have become 'insulin resistant'. Food has a major impact on blood sugar levels and whilst sugar is a major factor in high blood sugar levels it is not sugar that causes diabetes. The cause of diabetes is the insufficiency of insulin (Type I) or the ineffectiveness of insulin (Type II).

Most diabetics are very good at monitoring their blood sugar levels and understand the role of food and medication they have to undertake. They are usually on a diet recommended by their doctor.

Alcohol may increase the action of insulin, leading to hypoglycemia (low blood sugar), so people using insulin should avoid alcohol. Smoking may decrease insulin activity.[268] Smoking compounds the health problems associated with diabetes so people using insulin are cautioned to avoid smoking.

GLUCOSE INTOLERANCE

There are a great many people who have blood sugar problems who are not diabetic but have many symptoms. These clients we can help. Low blood sugar and high blood sugar have similar symptoms. Common symptoms of blood sugar imbalances are, irritability, fatigue — especially in the afternoons, constant thirst, lack of energy, the need for stimulants like coffee and tea, and dizziness if without food for more than six hours, headaches, blurred vision, excessive sweating, crying spells, fears and anxiety, palpitations and muscle cramps.

Chromium is often deficient in people who have ups and downs in their blood sugar levels. They need to be advised to eat little and often and never skip breakfast. By including protein and essential fatty acids into every meal and snack they have, will keep their blood sugar levels even resulting in more concentration, more productivity, more energy and generally feeling much better.

If we constantly eat sugar, the pancreas is constantly stimulated. If we eat any carbohydrate in refined form, white sugar, sweets, chocolate, white flour for example, digestion is rapid, and glucose enters the blood in a rush. In each case, the pancreas can over-react and produce too much insulin. Blood glucose then takes a rapid, uncomfortable drop, and may end up too low for normal functioning (hypoglycemia). If this over-stimulation happens too often, the pancreas becomes exhausted. Now, instead of too much insulin it produces too little. Too much glucose remains in the blood (hyperglycemia). In its most severe form, this condition becomes diabetes.

The regulation of blood glucose is a constant balancing act. The aim is to provide energy to the cells which need it, including the brain, and to make sure that unwanted glucose is not left circulating in the blood. If this balance is lost both physical and mental well being are in turn unbalanced. Low blood glucose and high blood glucose can have similar and wide-ranging effects.

Diet is of the utmost importance for people with out-of-control blood sugar. All refined carbohydrates must be removed from the diet. This includes honey and fruit juice. Research has shown that a whole-foods approach to diet, including fruit, vegetables, beans, nuts, and seeds is effective in reversing the insulin resistance seen in adult onset diabetes. They contain starch, which requires less insulin than simple sugars, high levels of fiber, natural antioxidants, essential fatty acids, and minerals.

Avoiding stress and taking regular exercise also help balance blood sugar levels.

RECOMMENDATIONS FOR GLUCOSE INTOLERANCE

DIET	A wholefood diet, with well-balanced meals containing food from all main food groups. Complete protein at every meal.
INCREASE	Fruit, vegetables, beans, lentils, nuts and seeds. Oily fish – sardines salmon, herring, tuna and mackerel.
DECREASE	All refined foods, especially those high in sugar, fizzy drinks, honey, citrus fruits, dried fruit, fruit juice, and alcohol. Avoid or cut down on cigarettes.
SUPERFOODS	Alfalfa, Algae, Barley Grass, Bee Pollen and bio-yoghurt.
SUPPLEMENTS	Multivitamin and mineral. Chromium GTF.
HERBALS	Siberian Ginseng – natural adaptogen
LIFESTYLE CHANGES	Frequent small meals, containing some protein. Always eat breakfast. Take regular exercise.

ENDOCRINE SYSTEM RULE NO 2

Never recommend fish oil capsules to diabetics
Some diabetics have experienced problems in glucose regulation

---

MENOPAUSE

The menopause is the cessation of the monthly female menstrual cycle. Women who have not had a period for a year are considered postmenopausal. Most commonly menopause takes place when a woman is in her late forties or early fifties. It is a perfectly natural part of being a woman, it is not a disease and cannot be prevented. Lifestyle and dietary changes can lead to the avoidance of many menopausal symptoms.

Exercise is important whatever age you are. Sedentary women are more likely to have moderate or severe hot flushes compared with women who exercise.[269] [270] In one trial, menopausal symptoms were reduced immediately after aerobic exercise.[271]

Many years ago researchers studied the effects of vitamin E in reducing symptoms of menopause. Most,[272] [273] [274] [275] [276] but not all studies found vitamin E to be helpful. 800ius per day are recommended of vitamin E for a trial period of at least three months to see if symptoms are reduced. If helpful, this amount may be continued.

Soybeans contain compounds called phytoestrogens, which can be described as weak oestrogens. Researchers have linked societies with high consumption of soy products to a low incidence of hot flushes during menopause.[277] As a result of many studies, nutritional therapists recommend that women experiencing menopausal symptoms eat tofu, soy milk, tempeh, roasted soy nuts, and other soy bean sources of phytoestrogens. Care must be made that the source is from non-genetically modified soybeans. Soy sauce contains very little phytoestrogen content, and processed foods made from soybean concentrates have low levels of phytoestrogen. Supplements containing isoflavones extracted from soy are commercially available, and flaxseed (as opposed to flaxseed oil) is also a good source of phytoestrogens.

Double blind studies support the usefulness of black cohosh for women with hot flushes associated with menopause.[278] A review of eight trials confirmed black cohosh to be both safe and effective.[279]

Sage may be of some benefit for women who are sweating excessively due to menopausal hot flushes during the day or at night.[280] It is believed this is because sage directly decreases production of sweat. This is based on traditional herbal prescribing and has been evaluated in clinical studies.

RECOMMENDATIONS FOR MENOPAUSE

DIET	A whole food approach to food where quality is more important than quantity. Plenty of fruits, vegetables, nuts and seeds with adequate essential fatty acids, low-fat protein, and plenty of water.
INCREASE	Fresh fruit, in particular berries: blackberries, strawberries, blueberries, and loganberries. Soybeans from unadulterated sources.
DECREASE	Everything refined – especially white bread and flour, confectionery, and alcohol.
SUPERFOODS	Soybeans and Flaxseed fiber
SUPPLEMENTS	A good all round multivitamin and mineral.
HERBALS	Black Cohosh Siberian Ginseng – corrects hormonal imbalance
LIFESTYLE CHANGES	Enjoy life to the full. weight bearing exercise is important at this time to support the skeletal system, but swimming and cycling are recommended too.

> ## ENDOCRINE SYSTEM RULE NO 3
> Eating little and often will keep blood sugar levels stable.
> Never skip breakfast and always have some complete protein with every meal or snack.

PROSTATE PROBLEMS

The prostate gland is a small gland that surrounds the neck of the bladder and urethra in males. It secretes a lubricating fluid, which forms the bulk of spermatic fluid and aids in the transport of sperm.

An enlarged prostate gland is more specifically known as benign prostatic hyperplasia and where natural therapies are the most effective. Prostatitis on the other hand, is an inflamed, swollen prostate usually due to infection, which may be acute or chronic and which should be referred to a GP.

The incidence of benign prostatic hyperplasia is estimated at 50 to 60 per cent of men between 40 and 59 years of age. Common symptoms of benign prostatic hyperplasia (BPH) are dysuria (painful urination), painful defecation, frequency of urination, inability to empty bladder fully, desire to urinate, incontinence of urine, possible fever, impotence, back pain and in some cases painful orgasm.

There are many possible causes: a diet too high in acidic foods (red meat, cheese, other dairy, protein foods, alcohol) excess tea, coffee and spices. and/or too little alkaline foods (green leafy vegetables, fruit,) and/or too little fibre, essential fatty acid and zinc deficiency. Other causes could be congestion, sluggish bowels, poor lymph and blood flow, toxicity of blood and poor abdominal tone. Lack of exercise and a sedentary occupation may also be factors.

European herbalists and naturopathic doctors have used saw palmetto for centuries for the treatment of BPH, but it was first used by Native Americans.. A three-year study in Germany found that 160mg of saw palmetto extract taken twice daily reduced nighttime urination in 73 per cent of patients and improved urinary flow rates significantly.[281]

Pygeum, an extract from the bark of the African tree, has been approved in Germany, France and Italy as a remedy for benign prostatic hypertrophy. Controlled studies published over the past twenty five years have shown that pygeum is safe and effective for individuals with BPH of moderate severity.[282] These studies have used 50–100mg of pygeum extract (standardized to contain 14 per cent triterpenes) twice per day. Pygeum relieves the symptoms of BPH. This herb contains three compounds that might help the prostate; pentacyclic triterpenoids, which have a diuretic action; phytosterols, which have anti-inflammatory activity; and ferulic acid which help rid the prostate of any cholesterol deposits that accompany BPH.

In another study, forty-five men with BPH received a supplement containing three amino acids (glycine, alanine, and glutamic acid) while forty other men with BPH were given a placebo. After three months, 66 per cent of the patients receiving the amino acid mixture showed reduced urinary urgency; 50 percent had less delay in starting urine flow; 46 per cent had less difficulty maintaining flow; and 43 percent had reduced frequency. In contrast, these improvements were reported by less than 15 per cent of the men who received the placebo. No side effects were observed.[283] Although it is not known how the amino acid combination works, it is believed to reduce the amount of swelling in prostate tissue.

Diet should be a high-fibre, non-citrus, alkaline-reacting diet, containing large amounts of raw green vegetables, essential fatty acids, and zinc. Zinc is paramount to effective treatment of BPH. Zinc deficiency becomes more prevalent with age and supplementation has been shown to reduce the size of the enlarged prostate and to reduce symptoms in the majority of patients. [284]

A good all-round multivitamin is highly recommended offering a minimum of 50mg of the B complex group of vitamins. Additionally, Starflower or Evening Primrose with no less than 15% GLA should be taken daily.

RECOMMENDATIONS FOR PROSTATE PROBLEMS

DIET	A whole food approach to food where quality is more important than quantity. Plenty of fruits, vegetables, nuts and seeds with adequate essential fatty acids, low-fat protein, and plenty of water.
INCREASE	Pumpkin seeds, oysters, oily fish – sardines salmon, herring, tuna and mackerel – up to three times per week.
DECREASE	Everything refined – especially white bread and flour, confectionery, and alcohol.
SUPERFOODS	Alfalfa, Medicinal mushrooms, bio-yoghurt and probiotics.
SUPPLEMENTS	Multivitamin and mineral. Evening Primrose Oil (GLA) Amino acids (alanine, glutamic acid and glycine). Zinc – liquid form for better absorption.
HERBALS	Pygeum Saw Palmetto – for every man over the age of 40. Don Quai – an adaptogen.
LIFESTYLE CHANGES	Learn how to manage stress. Take up relaxing hobbies and enjoy life.

THYROID DISORDERS

Hyperthyroidism covers a wide range of symptoms including insomnia, nervousness, weakness, sweating, over activity, sensitivity to heat, weight loss, tremor, and stare. Some of the main causes are vitamin A, E and B6 deficiency, liver damage, insufficient enzyme production to inactivate thyroid hormones, emotions and diet pills.[106]

However, thyroid deficiency is much more common and is referred to as **hypothyroidism**. Its symptoms also cover a wide range including fatigue, headaches, chronic or recurrent infection, eczema, psoriasis, acne, menstrual disorders, painful menstruation, depression, cold sensitivity, psychological problems and anaemia. Some of the main causes are iodine, vitamin E, vitamin A and zinc deficiencies. A history of taking diet pills, emotions and hereditary predisposition[106] are also causes of hypothyroidism.

The thyroid gland plays a key role in controlling the body's metabolic rate. It is in turn controlled directly by secretions from the pituitary and hypothalamus in the brain. The hypothalamus is affected greatly by strong emotions. Since the thyroid has a major effect on metabolism and the blood glucose level, it also has a strong effect on the mental state, causing mental depression, lethargy, fatigue, and psychosis. This may play a role in abnormal mental states in puberty, pregnancy, postpartum depression and menopause.

Iodine deficiency is probably the most common cause of hypothyroidism and this is easily corrected by consuming iodine-containing foods. Certain foods however, called goitrogens, actually hinder iodine utilisation and induce an iodine deficiency by combining with the iodine and making it unavailable to the thyroid. These include kale, cabbage, peanuts, soy flour, brussel sprouts, cauliflower, broccoli, radishes, mustard greens, kohlrabi, and turnips. I am not suggesting not to eat these foods, but rather that they are not to be eaten in excess. In general cooking inactivates these goitrogens. Good sources of iodine include saltwater fish, sea vegetables (kelp, dulse, arame, nori, kombu) and iodised salt.

The general treatment for thyroid disorders is based on a gentle stimulation of the thyroid through proper diet, food supplements and herbs to raise general vitality and assist in balancing the hormones. A daily multivitamin containing 50mg of B complex is usually recommended together with zinc 25mg daily taken in the evenings. Vitamin A up to 10,000ius daily is also recommended, as hypothyroid patients do not convert beta-carotene to vitamin A efficiently.

Desiccated thyroid, from which the thyroid hormones have been removed, is another way to increase thyroid hormone secretion. The idea here is that it supplies all the known nutrients needed to ensure proper functioning of the thyroid. These products are safe to use and are available in health food stores, but may not be suitable for strict vegetarians.

HOME TEST FOR THYROID DISORDERS:-

A useful home test for hypo or hyperthyroidism is the basal body temperature test as first suggested by Dr Broda Barns. Axillary temperature is taken for 10 minutes first thing in the morning. Average ranges are 97.8 to 98.2F. Temperatures below this range suggest hypothyroidism and those above hyperthyroidism. Women must take temperature on days 2 and 3 of the menstrual flow to get an accurate measurement. [114]

RECOMMENDATIONS FOR THYROID DISORDERS

DIET	A whole food approach to food where quality is more important than quantity. Plenty of fruits, vegetables, nuts and seeds with adequate essential fatty acids, low-fat protein, and plenty of water.
INCREASE	Saltwater fish, sea vegetables (kelp, dulse, arame, nori, kombu) iodised salt, mushrooms, watercress, seafood, egg yolks and wheat germ.
DECREASE	Vegetables from the brassica family: cabbage, broccoli and cauliflower should be decreased (but not avoided) together with corn, sweet potatoes, lima beans, and pearl millet (decreased but not avoided). Avoid everything refined – especially white bread and flour, confectionery, and alcohol.
SUPERFOODS	Spirulina, chorella and blue-green algae – rotate. Super sprouts, and bio-yoghurt. Watercress – acts as a tonic for regulating metabolism
SUPPLEMENTS	Vitamin A, Zinc, Desiccated thyroid, Selenium, B-complex
HERBALS	Garlic, preferably raw in salads, or as a capsule. Saw Palmetto – for every man over the age of 40. Don Quai – an adaptogen which increases circulation for better healing, prevents bleeding and strengthens and nourishes the glands. Black Cohosh – stimulates secretions of the liver, kidneys and lymph glands and expels mucous.
LIFESTYLE CHANGES	Avoid all chemicals – lead, aluminium and mercury.

GENERAL RECOMMENDATIONS FOR
THE ENDOCRINE SYSTEM

DIET **FOODS TO SUPPORT**	Broccoli is an excellent source of chromium, the trace mineral that assists the pancreas to work more efficiently and therefore increase insulin's efficiency, which has a knock on effect to regulate blood sugar. Other high chromium foods are brewers yeast, nuts, wheat cereals and mushrooms (*restrict broccoli for hypothyroidism*). Oily fish – sardines salmon, herring, tuna and mackerel.
FOODS TO AVOID	Everything refined – especially white bread and flour, confectionery, and alcohol.
SUPERFOODS	Spirulina, chorella and blue-green algae – rotate. Super sprouts, and bio-yoghurt. Watercress – acts as a tonic for regulating metabolism
SUPPLEMENTS	B complex Evening primrose oil, The antioxidant group of vitamins and the mineral selenium. Zinc and Magnesium.
HERBAL REMEDIES	Black Cohosh, Ginger Marshmallow, Don Quai Siberian Ginseng and Garlic.
LIFESTYLE CHANGES	Lose weight, as excess weight promotes insulin resistance and is generally unhealthy. Avoid all synthetic hormones. Avoid tampons (or buy sanitary wear specially prepared without bleach). Avoid all chemicals – lead, aluminium and mercury. Learn how to manage stress. Take up relaxing hobbies and enjoy life.

THE LYMPHATIC SYSTEM & IMMUNITY

What is the Lymphatic system?

The lymphatic/immune system consists of a fluid called lymph, vessels that transport the lymphatic fluid called lymphatic vessels (lymphatics), and a number of structures and organs that contain lymphatic tissue.

Main functions:

The lymphatic system has three main functions: to help us fight infection by identifying the body's enemies and, by filtering lymphatic fluid destroying the invading micro-organisms; in the distribution of fluids and nutrients around the body, especially protein molecules that are too large to pass back through the blood capillary walls and in absorbing the products of fat digestion from the villi of the small intestine.

What does the Lymphatic system actually do?

Specialised white blood cells known as lymphocytes are reproduced in the lymph nodes and when infection strikes, they generate antibodies to protect the body against subsequent infection. Therefore the lymphatic system plays an important part in the body's immune system.

The lymphatic system is important for the distribution of fluid and nutrients in the body, because it drains excess fluid from the tissue spaces and returns it to the blood via the lymphatic vessels and ducts. Protein molecules, which are too large to pass back through the capillary walls into the blood stream are especially important to be returned to the blood so are carried through the lymphatic system and returned via the lymphatic ducts.

The lymphatic system also plays an important role in absorbing the products of fat digestion from the villi of the small intestine. While the products of carbohydrate and protein digestion pass directly into the bloodstream, fats pass directly into the intestinal lymph vessels, known as lacteals.

Dietary influences affecting the lymphatic system

The lymphatic system, like all the other systems in the body relies heavily on an optimal intake of vitamins and minerals. We depend on our lymphatic system to provide antibodies when we need them and for this they particularly need vitamin B6. As all nutrients work synergistically, a deficiency in just this one vitamin could compromise our whole lymphatic and immune system. Deficiencies in iron, zinc, magnesium and selenium will all suppress immunity, as will deficiencies in vitamins A, B1, B2, B6, B12, folic acid, C and E.

What you eat can strongly influence the performance of white blood cells, the front-line warriors against infection and cancer. These are the neutrophils that engulf and kill bacteria (phagocytosis) and cancer cells, and the lymphocytes that include the T-cells , B-cells and natural killer (NK) cells. The B-cells produce antibodies to destroy foreign invaders such as viruses, bacteria, and tumor cells. T-cells direct many immune activities and produce two chemicals called interferon and interleukin that are essential in warding off infections and cancer. Natural killer cells are called the body's first line of defense against the development of cancer; they destroy cancer cells as well as virus-infected cells. There are now hundreds of research papers that document various foods and components of food that control the blood concentrations of white cells and their potency. Thus, fresh, good, nutritious food acts to stimulate and support the immune system. Whereas anti-nutrients, such as alcohol, lead, cadmium, and antibiotics can depress an immune system. The new classes of superfoods are especially beneficial for the immune system.

The most beneficial diet for the lymphatic system is basically the same as for all the systems in the body, which is whole food approach to food where quality is more important than quantity with abundant fruits and vegetables, low-fat protein, sufficient essential fatty acids and plenty of water. However, the emphasis should be placed on protein, because immune cells are produced rapidly during an infection, sufficient protein is essential. However, because protein uses up B6 in its metabolism, too much may in turn *suppress* the immune system, as we need the B6 to make the antibodies. A separate supplement of B6 and zinc is of particular benefit to boost the immune and lymphatic systems and well as a good all round multivitamin and mineral supplement containing all the antioxidants is imperative for a strong lymphatic and immune system.

Your immune strength needs certain nutrients to work efficiently. Deficiencies of vitamins A, B1, B2, B6, B12, folic acid, C and E suppress immunity, as do deficiencies of iron, zinc, magnesium and selenium.

Vitamins B1, B2 and B5 have mild immune-boosting effects compared to B6 as the production of antibodies, so critical in any infection, depends upon B6, as does T-cell function.

A good all round multivitamin and mineral taken every day will boost immune function. The antioxidants really come into their own when fighting off infections and in particular Vitamin C. If you are always suffering from frequent infections it may be worth considering taking an antioxidant. A good antioxidant supplement will include Vitamins A, C, E and the mineral Selenium.

COMMON DISORDERS
ALLERGIES

Allergies are responses mounted by the immune system to a particular food, inhalant, or chemical. The terms food sensitivity and food intolerance are general terms and are not usually associated to true allergic reactions, as although they often produce many unpleasant symptoms, they do not provoke the immediate reaction a true classical allergy does.

A true allergy is an IgE mediated reaction characterised by an immediate onset of symptoms usually within two hours. The reactions are intense, sudden and dramatic, proving extremely distressing for the patient and may even be life threatening.

Food intolerance on the other hand is IgG mediated and often characterised by delayed reactions occurring several hours, or even days, after digestion. Food intolerance (often referred to as sensitivity, hyper-sensitivity, delayed or false food allergy) are usually associated which chronic complaints such as migraine, eczema, asthma, childhood hyperactivity, irritable bowel syndrome and arthritis. There are many other conditions that may have their cause linked to food sensitivities and these include adult acne, rheumatoid arthritis, ADD (attention deficit disorder), yeast infection, colic, constipation, Crohn's disease, depression, diarrhoea, ear infections, and gallbladder attacks.

A common condition causing food intolerance is a leaky gut. These intolerances may or may not turn into full true allergies over time, as other factors are involved including heredity, an overly sensitive immune response, poor digestive function, excessive exposure to a limited number of foods, and the extent of the leakiness of the gut walls.

People often experience symptoms when foods, particularly protein foods which have been incompletely broken-down due to poor digestive function, pass through the digestive tract and into the small intestine to be absorbed. In normal circumstances, the protein molecules being too large to be absorbed would be passed through the system into the large bowel for excretion. However, with an excessively permeable gut (a leaky gut) the protein molecules are absorbed and the body reacts accordingly to something it perceives as 'foreign'. So for example, something you have eaten for years will suddenly give you uncomfortable symptoms. You think you know what the food is, but are convinced it couldn't be that food, for the simple reason that you *have* eaten it for years. So you continue to eat the offending food – and your symptoms persist. As the gut becomes more permeable, more and more food molecules are entering the body which otherwise would not. You will not be allergic to these foods, but will certainly be 'sensitive' or 'intolerant' to them. Once you have established the permeability of your gut and repaired it if necessary, you will be able to eat the food again with out getting the unpleasant symptoms.

Most people are therefore unaware that they are sensitive to foods because most only think of allergies as an immediate reaction, like hives or asthma attacks. Far more common are the 'false', 'masked' or 'delayed' reactions, which can occur up to 48 hours after ingesting the offending substance. Because the foods that we are sensitive to are often the foods that we eat every day, it is often extremely difficult to identify the offending food.

Rheumatoid arthritis may be linked to food allergies and sensitivities. In many people symptoms are made worse when they eat foods to which they are allergic or sensitive and made better by avoiding these foods. English researchers suggest that one-third of people with RA can control the disease completely through allergy elimination.[247] Finding and eliminating foods that trigger symptoms should be done with the help of a nutritional therapist experienced in allergies.

Unrecogised food allergy or sensitivity is a contributing factor in a significant number of asthmatic people and a link has been confirmed by double-blind research, particularly for nuts, peanuts, eggs and soy.[285]

More and more children are becoming hyperactive, delinquent and are being diagnosed with ADD – attention deficit disorder. ADD has been linked in studies to certain foods, inhalant allergens and food colours.[286] [287] [288] In a study of twenty children, their poor ability to concentrate and behaviour problems vanished when allergenic foods were removed from their diets.[289] More often than not if the children with these conditions don't have food allergies or sensitivities, then they do have either sugar imbalances, vitamins and minerals deficiencies (often zinc and B6 or niacin) or deficiencies of essential fatty acids. Once the offending foods or deficiencies have been identified, the children quickly respond and become manageable and learning improves.

The top offending food allergies and sensitivities in the UK today are wheat, dairy foods, citrus fruits, nuts, and tomatoes.

Some doctors report that food sensitivities may exacerbate gallbladder attacks in people who have gallstones. Preliminary research has found that foods most commonly reported to be triggers include eggs, pork and onion, though specific offending foods may vary considerably from person to person.[290]

Some and perhaps most people with Irritable Bowel Syndrome are sensitive to certain foods. People that have IBS often experience improvement when food sensitivities are discovered and those particular foods avoided. Tea is a common sensitivity for people with IBS.

Ionized air may also play a role in allergies. Research suggests that some allergy-provoking substances such as dust and pollen, have a positive electrical charge. Meanwhile, negative ions appear to counter-act the allergenic actions of these positively charged ions on respiratory tissues. Negative ions generally lead to favourable actions, and many individuals experience relief from their respiratory allergies.[120] Other allergy sufferers report considerable relief, with a few allergy reactions resolving completely, after negative ion therapy. The majority of allergy sufferers appear to be able to reduce reliance on other treatments (nutritional, biochemical or prescription) during negative ion therapy.

FOOD PHENOLICS

Food phenolics are natural flavourings, colourings and preservatives in foods. Many clients whose symptoms are due to the phenolic compounds are not allergic to them but are intolerant or sensitive to them. They are able to tolerate a limited amount of the phenolic, but if the intake exceeds this then symptoms occur. It appears that the tolerance level reduces the more symptoms occur, but that if the phenolic is avoided or the client is treated, the tolerance increases. For example, take a client with migraine who is sensitive to tyramine (a food phenolic). Some days he will take foods containing tyramine, but in low concentration and will not have a headache. On other days he will take the same foods in high concentration past his tolerance level and get a headache. If he avoids tyramine entirely for some months, or is desensitised, be will be able to take a level of tyramime which previously would have precipitated a headache. Tyramine is a common trigger for migraine and other headaches. It has been shown that some clients with migraine have a genetic deficiency of the enzyme which metabolises tyramine and an excessive intake will trigger an attack.

Tyramine is contained in: banana, bass, soya beans, beef, beer, cheese, cottage cheese, chicken, cocoa, chocolate, egg, oyster, pea, plum, pork, potato, sweet potato, prunes, raisins, spinach, tomato, walnut and yeast.

Take all these foods spread over say a ten-day period and the client may have no symptoms but taken over a two day period may result in a migraine attack.

Coumarin is one of the most common to cause problems and is unfortunately one of the most widespread phenolics. Apart from asthma, it can cause rhinitis, catarrh and other respiratory conditions. Coumarin is contained in: apple, banana, barley, beef, beer, beetroot, celery, cheese, cottage cheese, chicken, cocoa, chocolate, corn, egg, lemon, lettuce, lime, cow's milk, goat's milk, mutton, oats, pea, peanut, peppercorn, sweet potato, rice, tomato, tuna, turkey, wheat and yeast.

Again, all these foods taken over say a ten-day period may produce no reactions but taken over a two day period may result in an asthma attack.

There are many natural phenolics you may be sensitive to in excess and only an allergist will be able to identify them for you.

There are many tests available for identifying food intolerances and allergies. The most effective ones are the 'avoid and challenge' test and the elimination diets.

The 'avoid and challenge' test is a very simple test to check that if avoidance of a particular food leads to reduction in symptoms and reintroduction of that food leads to worsening of symptoms, then you have a sensitivity to that food. Bearing in mind that some foods may take 2 – 3 days to show a reaction the avoidance of that food has to be longer than that.

1. Choose one food or a food group to which you want to test (dairy products or wheat for example).
2. Completely avoid that food or food group for 14 days – the longer you avoid the food the more accurate the results will be.
3. At the end of the avoidance period (say day 15), sit is a quite place with no interruptions and take your resting pulse for 1 minute.

4. Then 'challenge' your body by eating more than usual of the food you are avoiding (a large glass of cow's milk if you are avoiding dairy).
5. Still siting quietly, re-take your pulse after 10, 30 and 60 minutes. If your pulse goes up by 10 points or if you have any noticeable symptoms within 48 hours you probably have an allergy or intolerance to this food. The symptoms are more important than the pulse, since some foods can raise the pulse without denoting an allergic reaction.

Do not carry out this test alone in case you have a strong reaction to the food you are testing. If you suspect you have food allergies or intolerances seek assistance from a nutritional therapist who will support you through the testing time.

LYMPHATIC SYSTEM & IMMUNITY
RULE NO 1

SIGNIFICANTLY REDUCE SUGAR INTAKE

Three ounces of sugar in **any** form, honey, fruit juice, sucrose, results in a 50% reduction in white cell activity for one to five hours!

RECOMMENDATIONS FOR FOOD SENSITIVITIES

DIET	A whole food approach to food where quality is more important than quantity. Plenty of fruits, vegetables, nuts and seeds with adequate essential fatty acids, low-fat protein, and plenty of water.
INCREASE	Unadulterated, organic, unpackaged food. You are less likely to have reactions to natural food (natural phenolics).
DECREASE	Everything refined — especially white bread and flour, confectionery, and alcohol and any food you suspect you may be sensitive to.
SUPERFOODS	Take care, as you may be sensitive to pollens, grasses or fungal foods, of which make up some of the superfoods.
SUPPLEMENTS	An all round multivitamin and mineral supplement with good levels of the antioxidant vitamins ACE with selenium.
HERBALS	The anti-histamine, antioxidant and anti-inflammatory actions of Quercetin make this a favourite herbal remedy for any allergy/sensitivity situation. It also protects the stomach from ulcer disease and gastric distress and strengthens capillary walls.
LIFESTYLE CHANGES	Identify possible sensitivities and employ the assistance of a nutritional therapist to assist you in your investigations. A positive determined approach will be needed to ascertain food allergies.

CANCER

Much conflicting advice has been written over the past few years regarding cancer but one aspect is now certain and that is diet has an

important part to play in the prevention and management of cancer –
especially the hormone dependent cancers.

There are many different types of cancers with different causes, and
most are caused by carcinogens (cancer causing agents) that have been
taken into the body and which have caused cell damage, often free
radical damage.

HORMONE DEPENDENT CANCERS

Breast, uterine and ovarian cancers are hormone dependent. An excess
of the female hormone oestrogen appears to encourage the growth of
hormone related cancers. Why is it that Japanese women are only one
fifth as likely to develop breast cancer as American and European
women? One answer is diet. A Japanese woman is likely to eat six times
more vitamin D (30mcg daily) from fatty fish than Western women,
giving them vital protection against breast cancer. The United
Kingdom RDA for Vitamin D is 5mcg and many women do not get
even this small amount. When Japanese women move to America or
anywhere where there is a more 'western' diet their breast cancer rates
creep up and eventually approach those of western women. So is it
something in the eastern diet that prevents cancer or something in the
western diet that promotes it?

Scientists will take a long time to give us precise answers but there is
already overwhelming evidence. Diets high in saturated fats, refined
sugars and alcohol are very harmful to human bodies, whereas diets
high in Essential Fatty Acids from fatty fish, rich in whole and
unrefined foods, and foods high in plant oestrogens, are highly
beneficial to human beings, especially against hormone related cancers.
Making small but significant changes in your diet could half your
chances of getting cancer.

The first thing to do is to eliminate all carcinogens from the diet. These
include cigarettes, heavy metals like cadmium, lead, aluminium and
mercury; saturated fats, sweeteners, alcohol and all synthetic hormones.

Then the immune system needs to be built up with good food and
dietary supplements.

RECOMMENDATIONS FOR CANCER

DIET	A whole food approach to food where quality is more important than quantity. Plenty of fruits, vegetables, nuts and seeds with adequate essential fatty acids, low-fat protein, and plenty of water.
INCREASE	Oily fish – sardines salmon, herring, tuna and mackerel. Fresh fruit and vegetables, including juices
DECREASE	Everything refined – especially white bread and flour, confectionery, alcohol, cigarettes, and sweeteners..
SUPERFOODS	Algae, Barley Grass, Bee Pollen, Cabbage, Medicinal mushrooms, Super sprouts.
SUPPLEMENTS	Multivitamin and mineral GLA from Evening Primrose Oil Antioxidant complex, Vitamin E, additional Selenium (check the amount already in the multi and antioxidant complex) Vitamin C – up to bowel tolerance.
HERBALS	Echinacea and Rhodiola
LIFESTYLE CHANGES	A positive approach to be taken. Seek support from family, friends and therapists. Lifestyle changes mostly to dietary intake. Only the best will do.

CANDIDA

Much has been written about this condition over the past years. The main symptoms of candida are frequent outbreaks of thrush and cystitis, a history of taking antibiotics, having been on the pill for many years and the main symptom of bloating. Bloating can also be a symptom of allergies so good diagnosis is important.

The usual bloating symptoms of candida are that when you wake up in the morning the stomach is 'flat' – as you eat through the day (bread, pasta, mushrooms, cheeses, refined foods like biscuits, cakes and sweets and yeast) then the stomach gradually extends as the candida is feeding also. By the end of the day, the stomach is so bloated that buttons have to be undone and clients feel extremely uncomfortable. Never assume that your client has candida. Advise of your suspicions and advise your client to see a clinical nutritionist to be given an anti-candida regime and encourage them that with patience and determination they can eliminate the problem. There are many 'short term' answers but for the long term and permanent relief a special regime is needed.

This regime usually follows a six-point plan.

1. An anti-candida diet for a minimum of two weeks to weaken the candida.
2. Taking a good multivitamin and mineral to support the client's immune system.
3. Taking a supplement to kill off the candida.
4. Reintroduce the probiotics to the gut.
5. Repair the gut wall.
6. Reintroduce the foods that were being avoided whilst on the diet.

The anti-candida diet is strict, and would include the following list of foods to avoid completely for the duration of the programme.

AVOID ALL — Sugar, and food containing sugar; that includes brown or white sugar, demarara, molasses, syrup, honey, sucrose, dextrose, lactose, maltose, fructose, confectionery, icing, marzipan, chocolate, ice-cream, desserts and puddings, cakes and biscuits, soft drinks including squash and all canned drinks, bottled ketchup, etc. Check all tins and packets for hidden sugar – even some frozen and tinned vegetables! (Malt is a form of sugar – see below).

Yeast, and all foods containing it or derived from it; that includes bread and even most pitta breads, food coated in bread crumbs, most pizza bases, Marmite, Vecon, Bovril, Oxo, etc., monosodium glutamate, citric acid, and vitamin tablets unless 'yeast free' is stated.

Refined grains, white flour, granary flour, which is white flour with malt and added grains), white rice, white pasta, cornflour, custard powder, cornflakes and cereals unless 'whole grain' is stated.

Malt and malted products some cereals (eg Weetabix), brown Ryvita, granary bread, malted drinks like Ovaltine, Horlicks and Caro.

Fermented products, alcoholic drinks, ginger beer, vinegar and all foods containing vinegar (ketchups, pickles, salad creams, baked beans) soy sauce.

Cow's milk and most milk products, including cream and cheese. (Cottage cheese and natural yogurt are allowed).

Fresh fruit, raw, stewed, made into jam, marmalade or juice. Pure fruit juice is pure fructose, and often very high in mould!

Dried fruit, including prunes and the dried fruit in muesli.

Nuts unless freshly cracked – especially peanuts and peanut butter, which support the growth of the mould.

Smoked or cured fish and meat, including ham, bacon, smoked mackerel, smoked salmon.

Preservatives, which are frequently derived from yeast and can introduce a chemical substance to the body. (NB sausages, even without preservatives, are high in white cereal and animal fat)

Mushrooms, tea and coffee, even decaffeinated, which still contains drugs, and hot spices as they irritate the lining of the intestine.

Whilst following the above and avoiding all the foods mentioned, you should concentrate your thoughts on the foods you can enjoy. If you focus on the food you can have rather than on the foods you cannot have, you will have a better chance of success.

ENJOY — Yeast free and soda bread, made with whole-wheat flour or other grains. Some bakers will make a batch for your freezer.

Rice Cakes, Oatcakes (malt free), original Ryvita (not brown, it's malted!) Ryvita with sesame seeds, wholemeal crispbreads (read the labels carefully).

Pastry made with wholemeal flour or other grains, and don't forget you can still have pancakes, dumplings and crumbles!

Soya milk (sugar free). You will quickly adapt to it on cereal, and when cooked with oats or rice it becomes really creamy.

Unhydrogenated margarine – Vitasieg is good. Some other brands contain citric acid, so should be avoided.

Natural yogurt any make will do, but it mustn't have fruit! Also, just because some say 'live' does not mean that the others are not! (all yoghurts are live)

Cottage cheese, avocados, and potatoes (cooked in many different ways).

Breakfast – home-made muesli with oatflakes and other whole grains mixed with seeds, and soaked in water or yoghurt, porridge made with water or Soya milk, sprinkled with cinnamon or nutmeg, egg with whole-wheat soda bread and Vitasieg; rice cakes with cottage cheese.

Salad — at least one plateful a day.

Main meals — but aim to eat less red meat. Most meat contains residues of hormones and antibiotics unless it is organically produced. Lamb, rabbit and poultry are less likely to be affected, and fish is quite safe from this form of pollution, though it does have other hazards! Experiment with more vegetarian meals – a pulse combined with a grain makes an excellent protein, e.g. bean and vegetable pie or crumble, lentil sauce with whole-wheat spaghetti. Have lightly steamed fresh vegetables or salad with every meal.

Herbs and mild spices – cinnamon, coriander, turmeric etc.

DRINKS *Hot* – Barleycup, Rooibosch tea, any other herb teas (avoid those which contain malt), hot water with a slice of lemon.

Cold – bottled mineral water, filtered tap water, tomato juice (no citric acid or vinegar) natural yoghurt with sparking water! Add some ice and lemon to your sparkling mineral water to make it look good as well as taste good! (As an alternative to bottled water, use a filter jug and then fizz the water in a soda-stream machine).

RECOMMENDATIONS FOR CANDIDA

DIET	Anti-Candida diet regime
INCREASE	Vegetables, low fat protein foods as above
DECREASE	Bread, mushrooms, fruit eaten alone, pasta, biscuits, fruit juices, refined foods, coke, coffee, tea.
SUPERFOODS	Broccoli, Cottage Cheese, Avocados, Alfalfa, Cabbage, Sprouted Seeds, Spirulina.
SUPPLEMENTS	Multivitamin and mineral daily Caprylic Acid. Probiotics.
HERBALS	Garlic.
LIFESTYLE CHANGES	Strict diet must be maintained. Once you are clear of candida you will feel like a new person and be able to enjoy life to the full – the wait will be worth it.

CELLULITE

Although many doctors still dismiss this condition as non-existent, it can be a very distressing condition for many women.

The common denominator for most women with cellulite is poor circulation and diet, poor elimination from the large bowel, poor lymphatic drainage and insufficient exercise. This results in the inefficient removal of the waste products of metabolism and toxins absorbed from the environment which in turn is a precondition for cellulite.

Cellulite is difficult to get rid of but not impossible. It takes a positive woman to rid herself of this unsightly condition but with determination it can be done. What does it take? Strict diet, daily skin brushing, a detoxification regime, profound lifestyle changes and regular aerobic exercise.

Initially a detoxification regime would be undertaken. This could last for up to ten days when little would be eaten except fruits and vegetables. This would then progress to a diet that would include small amounts of low protein foods with still abundant supplies of fruits, vegetables, nuts and seeds. At all stages of the programme you would undertake skin brushing. For this you would need a long handled natural bristle brush which can be obtained from chemists and health foods shops. Every day, you would brush your dry skin with the dry brush from the bottom of your body working upwards. You would brush towards the lymph glands which are situated all over the body with the main ones being located behind the knees, under the arms, the groin area, and around the neck area. You would bath or shower after the skin brushing. This is an excellent way to stimulate your lymphatic system and to encourage the toxins to be removed from your body.

In addition to all this you would be undertaking aerobic exercises at least three times per week. This would involve attending a class or by determined walking or jogging on your part. Too little will be ineffective. Lifestyle changes would have to be dramatic. No coffee, tea, chocolate or junk food of any description – ever! A tall order you may say, but the results would be a new you that is for sure! Don't try it alone. Get some help from a nutritional therapist who will help you with a specifically made programme to suit your current lifestyle.

You don't need to become boring and anti-social on a regime like this. It can be fun if you allow it.

RECOMMENDATIONS FOR CELLULITE

DIET	Initially a detoxification diet lasting 10 days followed by a 75 per cent all raw diet with sufficient protein and essential fatty acids.
INCREASE	Everything raw – fruits, vegetables taken alone and in juices, or very lightly steamed or baked (as in baked apples). Generous amounts of water.
DECREASE	Everything refined – especially all sugars, white bread and flour, confectionery, and alcohol
SUPERFOODS	Alfalfa, Algae, Barley Grass, Bee Pollen, Cabbage, Honey, liquorice, Medicinal mushrooms, Super sprouts, and Bio-yoghurt.
SUPPLEMENTS	A multivitamin and mineral complex.
HERBALS	Milk thistle (supports the liver in the detoxification process).
LIFESTYLE CHANGES	Daily skin brushing should become as regular as brushing your teeth. Aerobic exercise three times a week. Learning to say no to coffee, tea, chocolate, alcohol and anything that will clog the body up with toxins.

LYMPHATIC SYSTEM & IMMUNITY RULE NO 2
Skin Brushing on a daily basis is
an excellent way to improve lymphatic function

CHRONIC FATIGUE SYNDROME

A multi-faceted disease regarded with suspicion by many people in the medical establishment, CFS is very real to those suffering from it. This is a complex condition and one that is difficult even for doctors to diagnose. The International Chronic Fatigue Syndrome Study group says that for a positive diagnosis of CFS, fatigue must also be accompanied by four or more of the following symptoms:-

Symptoms associated with Chronic Fatigue Syndrome

Substantial impairment of short-term memory or concentration
Sore throat
Tender cervical or axillary lymph nodes
Muscle pain
Multi-joint pain without swelling or redness
Headaches of a new type, pattern or severity
Unrefreshing sleep
Post exertion malaise lasting more than 24 hours.

CFS is also defined as unexplained fatigue of greater than or equal to six months duration. Fatigue alone or prolonged fatigue (not CFS) is fatigue lasting from one to up to six months only.

Often ME and CFS are grouped together as one disease but according to the World Health Organisation the use of ME (myalgic encephalo-myelitis) as a term to encompass all forms of chronic fatigue is inaccurate and should be discouraged. Nevertheless, many CFS practitioners do recognise ME as a specific illness in a proportion of CFS sufferers. Symptoms are that of a post viral condition linked to exertion, impaired circulation and Central Nervous System involve-ment. It is probably fair to say that all patients with ME have CFS but not everyone with CFS has ME.

Complexities of diagnosis aside, it seems likely that nearly all cases of Chronic Fatigue Syndrome involve some kind of disruption of the immune response. Recommendations should therefore focus on boosting immune strength.

Many natural health experts believe Candida Albicans – a yeast infection of the intestines and bowel may also be partly to blame. Candida overgrowth is a significant factor for many people feeling exhausted. With such a multi-faceted disease, recommendation is neither simple nor straightforward. Simple but effective lifestyle changes are the first course of action. Reduce or eliminate caffeine, white sugars and flours and refined foods and alcohol and food additives. Encourage a well-balanced whole food diet and strongly recommend they visit a nutritionist. Other useful steps are positive thinking, a walk in fresh air and plenty of natural mineral water.

Other research suggests that CFS may be partially due to low adrenal function resulting from different stressors –(mental stress, physical stress, chemical stress and viral illness) impacting the normal communication between the hypothalamus in the brain, pituitary gland and adrenal glands.

Magnesium levels have been reported to be low in CFS sufferers. [291] Oral supplementation is usually adequate but sometimes injections are necessary.

Vitamin B12 deficiency can cause fatigue. Occasionally however, reports, even double bind, have shown that people who are not deficient in B12 nonetheless have increased energy following a series of vitamin B12 injections. Some sources in conventional medicine have discouraged such people from getting B12 injections despite evidence to the contrary.

Carnitine is required for energy production in the powerhouses of the cells (the mitochondria). There may be a problem in the mitochondria in people with CFS. Deficiency of carnitine has been seen in some CFS sufferers.[292] One gram of carnitine taken three times daily led to improvements in symptoms in a recent preliminary investigation.

Liquorice root is thought to help by stimulating and adrenal glands and blocking the breakdown of active cortisol in the body. One case study found that taking 2.5g of liquorice root daily led to a significant improvement in a patient severely affected with CFS. 6 – 8 weeks of 2.5g daily may therefore show beneficial results.

Siberian Ginseng may also be useful. As an adaptogen it is thought to allow the adrenal glands to function optimally when challenged by stress. Siberian ginseng also contains complex polysaccharides (complex sugar molecules) which lend the herb its immune-supporting properties. 10mg of Siberian ginseng three times a day have been shown to have increased numbers of T-lymphocyte immune cells.

Foods to increase for Chronic Fatigue Syndrome – The long chain polysaccharides found in the various medicinal mushrooms have been shown to be potent immune modulators, boosting the anti-viral activity of the host's immune system.

Tackling Chronic Fatigue Syndrome takes persistence and courage on the part of the sufferer and lots of encouragement from practitioners.

RECOMMENDATIONS FOR CHRONIC FATIGUE SYNDROME

DIET	A whole food approach to food where quality is more important than quantity. Plenty of fruits, vegetables, nuts and seeds with adequate essential fatty acids, low-fat protein, and plenty of water.
INCREASE	Green leafy vegetables for the magnesium content. Oily fish – sardines salmon, herring, tuna and mackerel. Fruit – to be used as snacks.
DECREASE	Stimulants such as tea, coffee, chocolate and alcohol.
SUPERFOODS	Medicinal mushrooms,
SUPPLEMENTS	Carnitine, B12 (sublingual), Magnesium Vitamin C up to 3g daily. Multivitamin and mineral and an antioxidant complex.
HERBALS	Siberian Ginseng, liquorice root,
LIFESTYLE CHANGES	Eat little and often. Exercise is important to prevent the worsening of fatigue

> # LYMPHATIC SYSTEM & IMMUNITY RULE NO 3
> **VACCINATIONS** – cause a one to two week **suppression** of the immune response. Always take a multivitamin one week before vaccinations and for two to three weeks after.

RHEUMATOID ARTHRITIS

Rheumatoid arthritis (RA) is a chronic inflammatory condition; it is an autoimmune disease in which the immune system attacks the joints and sometimes other parts of the body.

The onset of rheumatoid arthritis can be abrupt. The synovial membrane thickens and joints swell with redness and tenderness. Symmetrical joint involvement is common and may migrate from joint to joint.

There are several dietary changes that might be helpful for rheumatoid arthritis. The role of dietary fats in RA is complex but potentially important. In experimental animals that are susceptible to autoimmune disease, feeding a high-fat diet increases the severity of the disease.[246]

There is evidence that people with RA eat more fat, particularly animal fat than those without RA. In short-term studies, diets completely free of fat reportedly helped people with RA, however, since at least some dietary fat is essential for humans, the significance of this finding is not clear.

Rheumatoid arthritis may be linked to food allergies and sensitivities. In many people symptoms are made worse when they eat foods to which they are allergic or sensitive and made better by avoiding these foods. English researchers suggest that one-third of people with RA can control the disease completely through allergy elimination.[247] Finding and eliminating foods that trigger symptoms should be done with the help of a nutritional therapist experienced in allergies.

Although exercise may increase pain initially, gentle exercises help people with RA. Swimming, stretching or walking are recommended.

Vitamin E may be helpful in rheumatoid arthritis. The concentration of vitamin E has been found to be low in the joint fluid of individuals with rheumatoid arthritis. This reduction of vitamin E levels is believed to be caused by consumption of the vitamin during the inflammatory process. In a double blind study, approximately, 1,800ius per day of vitamin E was found to be of benefit.[248]

Research suggests that people with RA may be partially deficient in pantothenic acid B5. In one trial those with RA had less morning stiffness, disability and pain when they took 2,000mg of pantothenic acid per day.[249]

The relationship of copper to RA is complex. Copper acts as an anti-inflammatory agent because it is needed to activate superoxide dismutase, an enzyme that protects joints from inflammation. People with RA tend toward copper deficiency.[250] The *Journal of the American Medical Association* quoted one researcher as saying that while 'Regular aspirin had 6% the anti-inflammatory activity of [cortisone] . . . copper [added to aspirin] had 130% the activity.[251] Several copper compounds have been used successfully with RA, and a single blind study using copper bracelets reported surprisingly effective results. However, under certain circumstances, copper might actually increase inflammation in rheumatoid joints. Moreover, the most consistently effective form of copper, copper aspirinate (a combination of copper and aspirin) is not readily available.

Many double blind trials have shown that the omega-3 fatty acids in fish oil, called EPA and DHA, help relieve symptoms of RA. The effect results from the anti-inflammatory activity of fish oil. It can take many months before the results become evident.

Oils containing the omega-6 fatty acid gamma linolenic acid (GLA) such as borage oil, black current seed oil, and evening primrose oil (EPO) have also been reported to be effective in the treatment of RA. The most pronounced effects were seen with borage oil, however, that may have been due to the fact that larger amounts of GLA were used (1.4g per day). The results with EPO were conflicting and somewhat confusing possibly because the placebo used in these studies (olive oil) appeared to have an anti-inflammatory effect of its own. In a double blind study, positive results were seen when EPO was used in combination with fish oil.[252] GLA appears to be effective because it is converted in part to prostaglandin series 1, a compound known to have anti-inflammatory activity.

Preliminary research suggests that boron supplementation at 3–9mg per day may be beneficial, particularly in juvenile RA. However, more research on this is needed.

Many herbs too have been through clinical trials with successful results. These include Boswellia, Tumeric, and Ginger.

Boswellia is a traditional herbal remedy from the Indian system of Ayurvedic medicine, and has been investigated for its effects on arthritis. A double blind study using Boswellia found a beneficial effect on pain and stiffness, as well as improved joint function. Boswellia showed no negative effects in this study. The herb has a unique inflammatory action, much like the conventional non-steroidal anti-inflammatory drugs (NSAIDs) used by many for inflammatory conditions. But unlike NSAIDs, long term use of Boswellia is generally considered safe and does not lead to irritation or ulceration of the stomach.

Several published case studies of people with rheumatoid arthritis taking 6–50mg of fresh or powdered ginger per day indicated that ginger might be helpful.

Tumeric is a yellow spice that is often used to make brightly coloured curry dishes. The active principle is curcumin, a potent anti-inflammatory compound, which protects the against free radical damage.

RECOMMENDATIONS FOR
RHEUMATOID ARTHRITIS

DIET	A whole food approach to food where quality is more important than quantity. Plenty of fruits and vegetables, low-fat protein, and plenty of water.
INCREASE	Oily fish – sardines salmon, herring, tuna and mackerel. Avocados, watercress, parsley, celery, bananas, brown rice, soya milk.
DECREASE	Red meat, cheese, milk, all refined carbohydrates, especially sugar, citrus fruits, wheat, alcohol, fried foods. Foods of the nightshade family: tomatoes, eggplants, potatoes, peppers and tobacco.
SUPERFOODS	Alfalfa, Algae – especially spirulina, Bee Pollen, Super Sprouts
SUPPLEMENTS	Evening Primrose Oil, Fish Oils, a good multivitamin/mineral supplement containing at least 50mg of the B vitamins.
HERBALS	Boswellia, Ginger, Turmeric
LIFESTYLE CHANGES	Regular raw vegetable juice. Carrot and celery juice, Watercress, celery and parsley juice – for internal cleansing. Avoid taking drinks with meals. Skin brushing.

SKIN DISORDERS
ECZEMA

The term eczema literally means 'to boil over', and is a common skin condition characterised by an itchy, red rash. Many skin diseases cause somewhat similar rashes, so it is important to have the disease properly diagnosed before it can be treated.

Eczema can be triggered by allergies. Many children with eczema have food allergies, according to data from double blind research, so the first course of action would be to determine if allergies are a factor. If the trigger of the allergy can be identified, avoidance of the allergen can lead to significant improvement.

It has been reported that when heavy coffee drinkers with eczema avoided coffee their symptoms improve. In one particular trial, it was the coffee that was causing the problems, not the caffeine.

Researchers have reported that people with eczema do not have the normal ability to process fatty acids, which can result in deficiency of gamma-linolenic acid (GLA).[266] GLA is found in evening primrose oil (EPO), borage oil and black currant seed oil. Most double blind research has shown that EPO overcomes this block and is therefore useful in the treatment of eczema.

Ten grams of fish oil providing 1.8 grams of EPA (eicosapentaenoic acid) per day were given to a group of eczema sufferers in a double blind trial. After twelve weeks, those taking the fish oil experienced significant improvement.[267] According to the researchers, fish oil may be effective because it reduces levels of leukotriene B4, a substance that has been linked to eczema. The eczema-relieving effects of fish oil may require taking large amounts for at least twelve weeks.

Vitamin C has had good results with eczema. It is thought that vitamin C does not act on the eczema directly, but affects the immune system in a positive way, thereby improving the eczema. It is suggested that 80mg per day per 2.2 pounds of body weight would reduce symptoms. Talk to a nutritional therapist if you are concerned about exactly how much vitamin C to take.

Liquorice root used either internally or topically may help alleviate symptoms of eczema. A traditional Chinese herbal preparation, which included liquorice, has been successful in treating childhood and adult eczema in double blind studies. Topically, glycyrrhetinic acid, a constituent of liquorice root, reduces the inflammation and itching associated with eczema. Some doctors who use herbal medicine suggest using creams and ointments containing glycyrrhetinic acid three or four times per day. Liquorice may also be taken as a tincture in the amount of 2–5ml three times daily.

Other topical herbal preparations to consider based on traditional herbal medicine are chamomile, calendula, and chickweed creams. Chamomile and calendula have anti-inflammatory properties, while chickweed is historically used to reduce itching.

The treatment of eczema for children and adults differ tremendously. With adults an exclusion diet may be introduced to identify food allergens and to clean up the system, but with children exclusion diets are unsuitable. If eczema started just after the child was weaned, you should be particularly suspicious of recently introduced foods. Many new mothers introduce solid foods too soon into a baby's immature digestive system and this can result in a food sensitivity or intolerance. If a baby has eczema who is being breast fed, then the mother should be screened for food allergies and the mother can be put on an exclusion diet.

When weaning babies, start with foods that are unlikely to give an allergic reaction like vegetables. Then you can move down this specially prepared list of foods prepared by nutritional therapists who specialise in infant nutrition. Keep a diary of when foods were introduced. This may help at a later date if allergies arise.

Vegetables, Fruit (except oranges), Nuts and seeds, Pulses and beans, Rice, Meat, Oats, barley and rye, Oranges, Wheat, Mild products and finally Eggs.

LYMPHATIC SYSTEM & IMMUNITY RULE NO 4

Unlike the blood circulation that has the heart to pump the blood, the lymphatic system only has your muscles –
so daily exercise is *highly recommended* for a healthy lymphatic system.

RECOMMENDATIONS FOR EXCEMA

DIET	A whole food approach to food where quality is more important than quantity. Plenty of fruits and vegetables, low-fat protein, and plenty of water.
INCREASE	Oily fish – sardines salmon, herring, tuna and mackerel Fluid intake, fresh fruit and vegetables.
DECREASE	Coffee, wheat and dairy products, plus everything refined – especially white bread and flour, confectionery, and alcohol.
SUPERFOODS	Manuka Honey can be applied locally with a loose bandage for children or adults. Probiotics. Medicinal mushrooms, Super Sprouts, Alfalfa, Algae, Bee Pollen.
SUPPLEMENTS	Fish Oil (EPA/DHA). Vitamin C, Zinc.
HERBALS	Liquorice, Witch hazel, Calendula, Chamomile
LIFESTYLE CHANGES	Have any potential allergens identified.

PSORIASIS

Psoriasis is a common skin disorder that affects 2 – 4 per cent of the UK population, both men and women equally. It produces silvery, scaly plaques usually on the knees and elbows, but can be anywhere on the body including the scalp and nails.

Stress is one of the major causes, but hormonal changes, especially in women is also an indicator, as many women experience psoriasis for the first time when they become pregnant, during puberty or during the menopause.

The relationship of exclusion diets in bringing relief to many chronic diseases has long been of interest to nutritional therapists and psoriasis is no exception. With still no lasting cure from orthodox means, many psoriatics are seeking help and advice from nutritional therapists to see if their condition can be helped from the inside out.

In my own research project *Nutritional Treatment of Psoriasis – 1993* my colleagues and I set out to establish a creditable link between the ingestion of certain foods, their effect on the liver, and subsequent improvement or otherwise, of psoriasis. There have been numerous dietary approaches for psoriasis dating back many years but none have gained general acceptance in the management of this disease.[191.] The majority of these dietary approaches include supplementation with dietary fish oil, whilst others have concentrated on the content of saturated fats and/or protein consumed by the patients.

The results of the research papers have not provided clear and consistent answers. In part, this may reflect the complexity and the number of variables in such experiments, as not all can be controlled to the same degree. To achieve the aim of my own study changes had to be monitored in skin condition and general health using a nutritional approach only. We took a specific interest in cleansing and detoxifying the liver, with a view to lightening the burden of this vital organ – it is the function of the liver to remove aberrant chemicals and pathogens from the body.

Naturopathically it is believed that if an individual is given the opportunity to 'detoxify' their body, and their liver is allowed to function as it should, then they will have every opportunity of enjoying full health and an absence of skin complaints.

A diet was formulated for this study which had to be flexible, so as not to make it too difficult for the participants, yet it had to lighten the liver burden. This was the reason that alcohol and pork were the only two items strictly prohibited. However, simple sugars and certain other foods were also initially to be avoided.

Alcohol was to be avoided because it is one of the worst liver poisons, causing the degenerative condition called cirrhosis, fatal to so many heavy drinkers. It also inhibits the absorption of zinc, which is an essential nutrient for a healthy skin. Pork was to be avoided because, out of all the meats eaten in the UK today, pigs have the highest saturated fat levels. Saturated fat is a good storage medium for chemicals such as antibiotics and growth enhancing drugs used during intensive farming. Humans therefore ingest such drugs when eating pork or its derivative products, putting the liver under greater stress. The results of my own three-month study showed an 84 per cent improvement of skin condition, whereas 9.1 per cent had no change and 6.1per cent became worse.[192]

In larger studies, ingestion of alcohol appears to be a risk factor in psoriasis in men, but not women.[193,194] However, it should be strongly recommended that women as well as men should avoid alcohol.

Cayenne contains a resinous and pungent substance known as capsaicin. This chemical relieves pain and itching by depleting certain neurotransmitters from sensory nerves. In a double blind study, application of a capsaicin cream to the skin relieved both the itching and the skin lesions for psoriasis sufferers.[195]

Many nutritional therapists believe that sluggish liver function is a contributing factor in psoriasis, possibly explaining why milk thistle seeds, which promote normal liver function, can be beneficial to psoriasis sufferers. To understand how milk thistle helps the liver, we need to take a look at this essential organ and what it does.

The liver is the largest internal organ in the body, weighing between $2\frac{1}{2}$ and $3\frac{1}{2}$ lb. It must constantly renew itself by producing new cells. This extraordinary organ replaces its approximately 300 billion cells every six months. To perform its essential activity, the liver is comprised of about 100,000 individual lobules or wheel-shaped structures.

One of the many main functions of the liver is detoxification by converting or removing harmful substances that we introduce into the body – including drugs, alcohol, medicines, poisons, and synthetic hormones like HRT, the pill and growth hormones found in meat and poultry.

There have been many clinical studies using milk thistle in the treatment of psoriasis, with excellent results. The skin is also an organ of detoxification, and if the liver is working under par, then it shows in the skin, in all sorts of forms, including psoriasis.

The more efficient the liver is at detoxifying, the healthier a person will be. Milk thistle helps the liver protect itself from harmful substances by altering the cell walls. It also accelerates the rate of protein synthesis, which helps the liver renew itself by stimulating the growth of new cells to replace those that have been damaged or destroyed by disease.

As a dietary supplement milk thistle is one of the most effective liver strengthening products available. It is a remarkable age-old remedy that has been proved by modern science.

Psoriasis sufferers sometimes use psyllium husk powder since maintaining normal bowel health is believed to be important for managing psoriasis. Psyllium acts as a bulk forming laxative to cleanse the bowel and encourage normal elimination. It is important to maintain adequate water intake when using psyllium.

Burdock root is described as a blood purifier or alterative.[196] and believed to clear the bloodstream of toxins. It has been used both internally and externally for psoriasis. Traditional herbalists recommend 2 — 4ml of burdock root tincture per day. For the dried root preparation, in tablet or capsule form, the common amount to take is 1–2g three times per day. Many herbal preparations will combine burdock root with other herbs such as yellow dock, red clover or cleavers.

RECOMMENDATIONS FOR PSORIASIS

DIET	A natural diet of wholefoods. Choose organic whenever possible. Quality more important than quantity.
INCREASE	Fruits, vegetables, and plenty of bottled water.
DECREASE	Alcohol, pork, hard boiled eggs, refined foods of all kinds.
SUPERFOODS	Alfalfa, Algae, Barley Grass, Super Sprouts and yoghurt.
SUPPLEMENTS	Flax seed Fish Oils (EPA/DHA).
HERBALS	Milk Thistle, St. John's Wort, Rhodiola, and Cayenne.
LIFESTYLE CHANGES	Plenty of sunshine. Relaxing activities such as yoga, visualisation and meditation. Never eat under stressful conditions.

STRESS

Stress is one of the great damagers of the immune system.[115] [116] Stress results in stimulation of the sympathetic nervous system, the part of the nervous system responsible for the fight or flight response. Stress also results in suppression of the parasympathetic nervous system, the part of the nervous system responsible for bodily functions during periods of rest, relaxation and sleep. The immune system functions better when the parasympathetic is uppermost that is when we are resting, relaxing or sleeping than when we are fighting or fleeing. Normally the sympathetic and parasympathetic systems balance each other, but under continued stress, the balance is lost and the immune system suffers. The increased activation of the sympathetic nervous system results in increased secretion of adrenal gland hormones, especially the corticosteroids and catecholamines. These hormones inhibit white blood cell function, decrease the production of lymphocytes, and cause the thymus gland, the master gland of the immune system, to shrink. The result is a significant reduction in immune function. Only recently have researchers discovered that T and B cells contain receptors on their cell membranes for these stress-induced hormones, which helps explain the immune system's sensitivity to stress.[117]

Nearly every disease we know can be aggravated or even caused by stress. There is stress related hypoglycemia, headaches, colitis, ulcers, enuresis, fatigue, high blood pressure and a whole host of other conditions. No list of supplements will cure stress if the cause is primarily emotional or due to external conditions.

The best recommendation for stress is to identify the cause. This could be a work related problem or a relationship problem. Having discovered the cause, the client may need recommending to a suitable counsellor that deals with that particular problem. Stress comes in many guises. There is physical stress, chemical stress, emotional stress, spiritual stress, and mental stress to name but a few.

LYMPHATIC SYSTEM & IMMUNITY RULE NO 5

HEAVY METALS – mercury (from amalgam fillings), cadmium (from other people's cigarette smoke and lead inhibit the formation of antibodies and reduce the bacteria-killing ability of white cells.
If you are susceptible to heavy metals –
the antioxidants (Vitamins A,C,E and the mineral Selenium) will help protect you.

RECOMMENDATIONS FOR STRESS

DIET	A whole food approach to food where quality is more important than quantity. Plenty of fruits, vegetables, nuts and seeds with adequate essential fatty acids, low-fat protein, and plenty of water.
INCREASE	Slow releasing carbohydrates, fruit and vegetables, oily fish.
DECREASE	Meat, high saturated fat foods, alcohol, and sugar of all types
SUPERFOODS	Alfalfa, Algae, Barley Grass, Bee Pollen, Cabbage, Manuka honey, Medicinal mushrooms, Super sprouts and Bio-yoghurt.
SUPPLEMENTS	Multivitamin and Mineral, B Complex (checking amounts with the multi) up to 50mg of all the B complex in total. Vitamin C up to 3g daily.
HERBALS	Echinacea, Garlic, Ginkgo Biloba, Rhodiola, Valerian.
LIFESTYLE CHANGES	Take up yoga, meditation, gentle regular exercise like walking or swimming. Learn how to deal with stress. Take time out for yourself and make it a priority.

VIRUSES –
THE HERPES SIMPLEX VIRUS 1 (COLD SORES)
THE HERPES SIMPLEX VIRUS 2 (GENITAL HERPES)

If you have ever had a cold sore then it was the Herpes Simplex virus that was responsible. Although the virus lies dormant in 90% of us, diet may well determine whether the virus becomes reactivated and explodes into herpes symptoms. Shingles, genital blisters, and Epstein-Barr disease are the same virus.

Much work was done on this virus in the 1950's and it was discovered that amino acids found in food could either stifle or encourage the growth of the herpes virus. Adding the amino acid arginine to the herpes virus in cell cultures made it grow like crazy. Adding the amino acid lysine halted the growth and spread of herpes viruses in cells.

A mere 55g (2ozs) of peanuts or chocolate is enough to cause an outbreak, especially if the diet was lacking in lysine. Lysine is found in milk, meat, and soya beans. It's not just the amount that is important but the balance between arginine and lysine in foods. Almonds, brazil nuts, cashews, hazelnuts, peanuts, pecans, walnuts, chocolate, Brussel sprouts and gelatin all have a high ratio of arginine to lysine and should therefore be avoided at the start of an outbreak.

If you cannot control your cold sore outbreaks by diet then you could consider taking a supplement of lysine. 500mg twice a day until the infection is under control.

LYMPHATIC SYSTEM & IMMUNITY RULE NO 6

Hydrotherapy – professional hot and cold water treatments undertaken at health spas
increases circulation to blood and lymph,
removes internal congestion and improves tissue vitality and nutrition.
A beneficial treatment for the lymphatic system.

RECOMMENDATIONS FOR VIRUSES

DIET	A light diet of high-energy natural foods, raw or lightly cooked. Include protein, as this is needed to make antibodies.
INCREASE	Foods high in vitamins A, B complex C and zinc should be increased as well as increased fluid intake (especially water).
DECREASE	Salt, and mucus forming and fatty foods such as milk, eggs and meat.
SUPERFOODS	Medicinal mushrooms, Super Sprouts, Bee Pollen, Spirulina, Chlorella and Blue-Green Algae (rotate every four weeks). Cabbage – especially the water is has been cooked in.
SUPPLEMENTS	Antioxidant complex containing A,C,E and Selenium Zinc and the amino acid lysine.
HERBALS	Aloe Vera, Grapefruit seed extract (a natural antibiotic) Ginger, Garlic, echinacea and Cat's Claw tea (an acquired taste but very beneficial).
LIFESTYLE CHANGES	Keep warm and get plenty of rest. The immune system works better in a warm environment. If you are not better within 5 days seek the advice of your doctor.

GENERAL RECOMMENDATIONS FOR THE LYMPHATIC SYSTEM & IMMUNITY

DIET **FOODS TO SUPPORT**	A whole food approach to food where quality is more important than quantity. Plenty of fruits and vegetables, nuts and seeds, low-fat protein, and plenty of water. Oily fish – sardines salmon, herring, tuna and mackerel. Increased fluid intake.
FOODS TO AVOID	Alcohol, pork, hard-boiled eggs, refined foods of all kinds especially white bread, flour and confectionery.
SUPERFOODS	Alfalfa, Algae, Barley Grass, Super Sprouts Probiotics, Medicinal mushrooms, Super Sprouts, Bee Pollen and yoghurt. Manuka Honey can be applied locally to any skin condition with a loose bandage for children or adults.
SUPPLEMENTS	Fish Oil (EPA/DHA). Vitamin C Zinc, Flax seed. Antioxidant complex.
HERBAL REMEDIES	Liquorice, Witch hazel, Calendula, Chamomile Milk Thistle, St John's Wort, Rhodiola, Cayenne.
LIFESTYLE CHANGES	Skin Brushing Hot and Cold Sitz Baths Regular daily aerobic exercise Learning to say no to coffee, tea, chocolate, alcohol and anything that will clog the body up with toxins.

THE MUSCULAR SYSTEM

What is the Muscular system?

The term *muscle tissue* refers to all the contractile tissues of the body; skeletal, cardiac and smooth muscle. Cardiac muscle tissue is located in the heart and is therefore considered part of the cardiovascular system. Smooth muscle tissue of the intestine is part of the digestive system, whereas smooth muscle tissue of the urinary bladder is part of the urinary system. The *muscular system,* however, refers only to skeletal muscles, the muscles that are under our voluntary control.

Main function

The main function of the muscular system is that of movement.

What does the Muscular system actually do?

There are nearly 700 skeletal muscles in the body. Skeletal muscles produce movements by exerting force on tendons, which in turn pull on bones or other structures such as the skin. Most muscles cross at least one joint and are attached to the articulating bones that form the joint. When such a muscle contracts it draws one articulating bone toward the other.

Dietary influences affecting the muscular system

Probably the most influencing factor to the muscular system is water. Muscles are 75 per cent water and a loss of only 3 per cent of this water causes a 10 per cent drop in strength and an 8 per cent loss of speed. Carbohydrates too are essential with regard to the muscular system as carbohydrates provide the necessary fuel. This is why many athletes will 'carbohydrate load' before an event. Protein is important but should be kept to a minimum. Increasing protein does not improve athletic performance, and whilst fat has little role to play, the essential fatty acids must not be overlooked.

COMMON DISORDERS
CRAMP

Cramp is a common and painful condition that is caused by the prolonged contraction of a muscle. Cramps normally last for only a few seconds and can be put down to things such as poor posture, stress or tiredness. Sometimes a cramp will occur just after exercise because of a build up of lactic acid in the muscles. Many people suffer from night cramps will usually be relieved by massage or stretching. Cramps are usually caused by impaired blood supply to the muscles and supplements that promote blood flow often reduce the frequency of attacks.

Chamomile has a high content of calcium and magnesium and also contains potassium, iron, manganese, zinc and vitamin A. It makes a pleasant tea and is excellent for menstrual cramps.

Wild yam is useful for cramps in the region of the uterus during the later stages of pregnancy. It will relax and soothe muscles and nerves.

Muscle cramps can be quite debilitating but can respond to vitamin E, B6, calcium and magnesium.

MUSCULAR SYSTEM RULE NO 1
ALWAYS Warm-up before exercise
ALWAYS cool-down muscles after exercise

RECOMMENDATIONS FOR CRAMP

DIET	A whole food approach to food where quality is more important than quantity. Plenty of fruits, vegetables, nuts and seeds with adequate essential fatty acids, low-fat protein, and plenty of water.
INCREASE	Green leafy vegetables, oily fish at least three times a week
DECREASE	All denatured food, all stimulants such as tea, coffee, chocolate, cigarettes and alcohol. All refined foods such as white bread and flour and all synthetic colourings and flavourings.
SUPERFOODS	Algae, Bio-yoghurt, Medicinal mushrooms.
SUPPLEMENTS	Magnesium and calcium supplement. Co-Q-10, Vitamin E, B-complex supplement with B6 Antioxidant formula.
HERBALS	Chamomile, Wild yam.
LIFESTYLE CHANGES	Be sure to warm up and cool down before and after events. Cramp can be caused by dehydration, so don't forget the fluid intake.

FYBROMYALGIA

Fibromyalgia is a health condition that involves muscular pain and stiffness, which is usually considered to be a form of arthritis. However, because it is characterised by a number of tender points all over the body in specific muscles, it is more of a muscular energy disorder than arthritis.

Anti-inflammatories are often recommended as in Evening Primrose oil and in some cases these help, but the problems appear to be more with the energy the muscles are not providing than an inflammation problem. There are natural pain killers than can be recommended.

It is a complex syndrome with no known cause or cure. Some of the most common symptoms of this syndrome are: aches and pains in the muscles, tendons and ligaments, fatigue and restlessness, muscle spasms, stiffness, headaches and paresthesia (tingly, prickly sensations), sleep disorders, constant fatigue and a depressed immune function.

Low-intensity exercise may improve fibromyalgia symptoms. Patients who exercise regularly have been reported to suffer less severe symptoms than those who remain sedentary.[95][97][98]

Stress is believed by some researchers to be capable of exacerbating symptoms. Stress-reduction techniques such as mediation have also proven helpful in preliminary research.[93] As stress uses up magnesium, there is a need for magnesium supplementation. A special form of magnesium called magnesium malate, is often recommended for fibromyalgia sufferers.

Acupuncture has significantly improved symptoms in several trials studying people with fibromyalgia.[94]

MUSCULAR SYSTEM RULE NO 2
Muscles at 75% water
loss of only 3 per cent of this water causes a 10 per cent drop in strength and an 8 per cent loss of speed.
DRINK AT LEAST ONE LITRE OF WATER EVERY DAY

RECOMMENDATIONS FOR FIBROMYALGIA

DIET	A whole food approach to food where quality is more important than quantity. Plenty of fruits, vegetables, nuts and seeds with adequate essential fatty acids, low-fat protein, and plenty of water.
INCREASE	Green leafy vegetables and all fruits, nuts, seeds and low fat protein like free-range chicken and turkey. Oily fish — sardines salmon, herring, tuna and mackerel.
DECREASE	Cigarettes, alcohol, all refined foods, all anti-nutrients. Be aware of heavy metals, such as lead, cadmium, aluminium and mercury and avoid contact.
SUPERFOODS	Alfalfa, Algae, Barley Grass, Bee Pollen, Medicinal mushrooms, Super sprouts and bio-yoghurt.
SUPPLEMENTS	Magnesium malate. Fish oils and GLA, Antioxidant complex and a B-complex with at least 50mg of all the B vitamins.
HERBALS	2g liquorice root three times per day for six to eight weeks, Boswellia, applied as a cream has been beneficial. Rhodiola
LIFESTYLE CHANGES	Regular exercise but of the low-intensity type. Investigate an acupuncture treatment. Identify any food allergens that may be involved with the symptoms.

INJURY

Muscle injuries such as tears and strains are extremely common especially in athletes and people who engage in regular intensive training. Muscles need to be continually worked if they are to maintain their size and strength. In 1991 the space shuttle Colombia was launched for a nine day mission dedicated, among other things, to researching the physiological changes bought on by weightlessness. The crew experienced a 25% loss in muscle mass within 10 days – perfectly illustrating the importance of keeping muscles stimulated.

Regular weight bearing exercise is essential to maintain good muscle mass. Weight bearing exercise is walking, running jumping rope, not swimming, cycling or using a trampoline, which are all aerobic activities.

Prolonged exercise may result in muscles being broken down into amino acids to provide fuel for the body. Furthermore the health of the muscle tissue may be effected by wear and tear. To help maintain muscle structure people who engage in intense, long-duration activities may find that an amino acid complex supplement helps to promote regeneration of muscle tissue.

MUSCULAR SYSTEM RULE NO 3

In injury follow the **R I C E** principle.
Rest, Ice, Compression and Elevation

RECOMMENDATIONS FOR INJURY

DIET	A whole food approach to food where quality is more important than quantity. Plenty of fruits, vegetables, nuts and seeds with adequate essential fatty acids, and plenty of water. Complete protein is of importance for injury to help repair damage. Choose good quality protein like oily fish, free range chicken, turkey, free-range eggs.
INCREASE	Green leafy vegetables and spring water. Good quality, low fat protein.
DECREASE	Everything refined – especially white bread and flour, confectionery, and alcohol
SUPERFOODS	Spirulina, Medicinal mushrooms, Bee Pollen
SUPPLEMENTS	Amino Acid complex. Antioxidants Multivitamin and mineral Magnesium and Calcium.
HERBALS	Echinacea, Rhodiola, Ginkgo Biloba
LIFESTYLE CHANGES	Never forget to warm up and cool down. Regular massage is highly beneficial.

STRAINS & SPRAINS

A sprain is the forcible wrenching or twisting of a joint with partial rupture or other injury to its attachments without luxation. It occurs when the attachments are stressed beyond their normal capacity. There may be damage to the associated blood vessels, muscles, tendons, ligaments or nerves. A sprain is more serious than a strain which is the over stretching of a muscle. Severe sprains may be so painful that the joint cannot be moved. There is considerable swelling and pain may occur owing to underlying haemorrhage from ruptured blood vessels.

The ankle joint is most often sprained; the low back area is another frequent location for sprains.

RECOMMENDATIONS FOR STRAINS

DIET	None specifically. A well-balanced diet covering all the main food group; carbohydrates, essential fatty acids, and proteins. Good quality complete protein is needed for repair and renewal in the body so ensure you are getting enough.
INCREASE	Green leafy vegetables. Juicing is good in time of recovery. Experiment – carrot and apple, celery and apple, apple with a little lemon. All detoxifying and cleansing to aid healing.
DECREASE	Alcohol, cigarettes, all refined foods, junk food, chocolate, tea and coffee.
SUPERFOODS	Spirulina, Medicinal mushrooms, Bee Pollen
SUPPLEMENTS	Amino Acid complex. Antioxidants, Multivitamin and mineral Magnesium and Calcium.
HERBALS	Echinacea, Rhodiola, Ginkgo Biloba
LIFESTYLE CHANGES	Resting the injury is the only way to get back on your feet quickly. Ice may be helpful to reduce inflammation, taping the injury may be appropriate and elevation of the injured part.

GENERAL RECOMMENDATIONS FOR
THE MUSCULAR SYSTEM

DIET **FOODS TO SUPPORT**	Eat plenty of complete carbohydrates such as whole grains, fruit, vegetables, beans, lentils and jacket potatoes. Add some protein to your food such as low fat chicken, turkey, nuts and seeds. Drink plenty of water – but not carbonated water – unless it is natural – before, during and after events if you are an athlete.
FOODS TO AVOID	Too much protein and a diet high in unrefined foods.
SUPERFOODS	Alfalfa, Spirulina, Chorella and blue-green algae – rotated each month. Barley Grass, Bee Pollen, Cabbage, Manuka honey, Liquorice, Medicinal mushrooms, Super sprouts and Bio-yoghurt.
SUPPLEMENTS	Magnesium Vitamin E L-arginine and L-ornithine Amino Acid complex for serious athletes BCAA – Branched Chain Amino Acids. Co-Q-10
HERBAL REMEDIES	Ginger Ginkgo Biloba Garlic Liquorice Siberian Ginseng.
LIFESTYLE CHANGES	Take nutrition seriously. Whether you are an athlete or a housewife, the difference between coming first or second or the difference between getting out of bed in the morning or not, may depend on your overall dietary habits.

THE NERVOUS SYSTEM

What is the Nervous system?

The Central Nervous System (CNS) is the control center for the entire nervous system and consists of the brain and spinal cord.

The Peripheral Nervous System (PNS) regulates the processes, in the form of nerves which connect the brain and spinal cord with receptors, like muscles and glands. The Peripheral Nervous System can then be divided into an afferent system and an efferent system. The afferent system consists of nerve cells that convey information *from* receptors to the CNS. The efferent system consists of nerve cells that convey information from the CNS *to* muscles and glands.

Main function

The overall function of the nervous system is to collect information about the external conditions in relation to the body's external state, to analyse this information, and to initiate appropriate responses to satisfy certain needs.

The principal cells of the nervous system are known as neurons. Neurons are highly specialised for nerve impulse conduction and for all special functions attributed to the nervous system: thinking, controlling muscle activity, and regulating glands. The other principal kind of cells found in the nervous system are called neuroglia. The neuroglia serve as a special supporting and protective component of the nervous system.

What does the Nervous system actually do?

All body sensations must be relayed from receptors to the central nervous system if they are to be interpreted and acted upon. The majority of nerve impulses that stimulate muscles to contract and glands to secrete must also originate in the central nervous system. The main sensations are cold, heat, pain, and pressure.

Dietary influences affecting the nervous system

As with all systems of the body, diet plays an important role in the nervous system. This is one system of the body we should all be concerned about, as dementia and other degenerative diseases of the brain are increasing and once these diseases develop, they may not be reversible. At such a time we are limited to improving function as best we can and limiting further degeneration. Obviously prevention is the best approach. A considerable amount of research shows that these degenerations are caused primarily by three factors: poor blood supply to the brain, nutritional deficiencies and brain-specific toxins- all of which are controllable. The irritation or inflammation of nerves may be caused by anemia, B1 deficiency or B12 neuropathy. Alcoholism and diabetes are also associated with nerve disorders.

COMMON DISORDERS
ANXIETY

Anxiety describes any feeling of worry or dread usually about potential events that may or may not happen. Some anxiety about stressful events is normal, however, in some people anxiety interferes with the ability to function. Severe anxiety usually lasts more than six months though it may not be a problem every day. Physical symptoms can sometimes result in fatigue, insomnia and irritability. Nutritional and natural therapies can be one part of the approach for helping relieve moderate anxiety.

Reducing exposure to stressful situations can help decrease anxiety. In some cases medication counselling or group therapy can facilitate this process.[151]

All sources of caffeine should be avoided including tea, coffee, chocolate, caffeinated drinks and caffeine containing medications. People with high levels of anxiety appear to be more susceptible to the actions of caffeine.[152]

For mild anxiety magnesium may be relaxing[153.] Typically 200–300mg of magnesium taken two to three times a day. Additionally many nutritional therapists recommend soaking in a hot bath containing 1–2 cups of magnesium sulphate crystals (such as Epsom salts) for fifteen to twenty minutes. Inositol has been used to help people with anxiety accompanied with panic attacks. Up to 4 grams three times per day has been reported to control such attacks in one double-blind trial.[154] Vitamin B3 as niacinamide may be beneficial. It has been shown in animals to work in the brain in ways similar to drugs such as Valium®, which are used to treat anxiety.[155] A reasonable amount of niacinamide (not niacin) to take for anxiety according to some doctors of natural medicine is up to 500mgs four times per day.

The herbal remedy that has been studied extensively in connection with anxiety is Kava Kava.[156] A study taken over a six week period showed Kava Kava to be just as effective as benzodiazepines.[157] St. John's Wort is probably most well known herb for the treatment of mild depression but it has also been reported in at least one well-known double-blind study to reduce anxiety.[158]

An old folk remedy for anxiety particularly when it causes insomnia is chamomile tea. There is evidence from test tube studies that chamomile tea contains compounds with a calming action.[159.] One cup of tea is taken three or more times per day. The chamomile tea should be drunk as strong as possible and if made with a tincture will be more effective than shop bought tea-bags. For anxious children put the tea mixture into the bath water. This is also beneficial for children and adults with eczema.

NERVOUS SYSTEM RULE NO 1

Prevention is better than cure – Look after your brain cells **NOW** by improving nutritional status.

RECOMMENDATIONS FOR ANXIETY

DIET	A whole food with meals containing all main food groups, especially small regular amounts of low fat protein foods.
INCREASE	Green leafy vegetables, fruits and whole foods.
DECREASE	Coffee, tea, chocolate and all fizzy drinks.
SUPERFOODS	Alfalfa, Algae, Super Sprouts, and Bee Pollen
SUPPLEMENTS	Multivitamin and mineral containing 50mg of the B vitamins (this will also contain sufficient magnesium)
HERBALS	Kava Kava, St. John's Wort and Valerian.
LIFESTYLE CHANGES	Reduce stress levels, take up yoga, meditation or visualisation.

HEADACHES

Some kinds of headaches such as those caused by hangovers or not enough sleep, are easily diagnosed and treated by drinking lots of water and catching up on sleep as soon as possible. Other types of headache tend to fall into three main categories: tension-type headaches, migraines and cluster headaches. Tension headaches are generally thought to be caused by the tightening of the muscles of the scalp and face, usually as a result of stress or bad posture, and can last for days or even weeks.

Migraines are typically characterised by sudden severe pain on one side of the head, nausea or vomiting and sensitivity to light, sound and odor. They are generally disabling for several hours or more.

Cluster headaches are quite rare, cause intense pain behind one eye and may wake the sufferer nightly for periods of weeks or months.

Diet can play an important part regarding headaches. It may be that the client is consuming too much of one type of food such as wheat, cheese, or other type of dairy food and may have an intolerance to this food resulting in headaches. The simple home allergy test referred to under 'Allergies' in the Immune System chapter of this book may shed some light if the culprit is in fact food.

RECOMMENDATIONS FOR HEADACHES

DIET	Low protein diets are recommended for headache sufferers. That is good quality low fat protein like free-range chicken, turkey, fish and free-range eggs.
INCREASE	Complex carbohydrates and low fat protein foods.
DECREASE	All refined foods, salt and dairy foods
SUPERFOODS	Super Sprouts, Medicinal Mushrooms and Alfalfa
SUPPLEMENTS	B-Complex (B2 in particular), Fish Oils, Magnesium
HERBALS	Feverfew, Ginger
LIFESTYLE CHANGES	Identify food allergies or intolerances, and stop smoking.

NERVOUS SYSTEM RULE NO 2

Ginkgo Biloba is the oldest, most effective and most researched herb for helping the brain

---

INSOMNIA

The ability to get a good night's sleep can result from waking up in the middle of the night and having trouble getting back to sleep as well as having a hard time of getting to sleep in the first place. Insomnia can be a temporary, occasional; or a chronic problem.

Caffeine is a stimulant.[160] The effects of caffeine last up to twenty hours,[161] so some people will have disturbed sleep patterns even when the last cup of coffee was in the morning. Besides regular coffee, black and green tea, cola, chocolate some soft drinks and OTC (over the counter) pharmaceuticals also contain caffeine.

Nutritional therapists will sometimes recommend eating a high carbohydrate filler before bedtime such as a slice of bread or some crackers. Eating carbohydrates can significantly increase serotonin levels in the body,[162] and the hormone serotonin is known to reduce anxiety and promote sleep.

Insomnia can be triggered by psychological stress. Dealing with that stress through counselling or other techniques may be the answer to a better night's rest. Psychological intervention has helped in many studies.[163]

A steady sleeping and eating schedule combined with caffeine avoidance and counselling sessions using behavioral therapy has reduced insomnia for some people, as has listening to relaxation tapes.[164] Melatonin, is a natural hormone that regulates the human biological clock and the body produces less melatonin with advancing age, which may explain why elderly people often have difficulty in sleeping [165.] Melatonin supplements are not available in the UK but are freely available in the USA.

There are many herbal remedies used for insomnia. The most reliable according to studies is valerian. Valerian root makes getting to sleep easier and induces deep sleep and dreaming. Valerian will not cause a morning hangover, a side-effect common to prescription sleeping drugs, and melatonin in some individuals.[166,167] A concentrated valerian root supplement in the amount of 300–400mgs can be taken 30 minutes before bedtime.

One German study compared the effect of a combination product containing an extract of valerian root (320mg at bedtime) and extract of lemon balm (*Melissa officinalis*) with the sleeping drug Halcion®. After monitored sleep for nine nights the herbal duo matched Halcion® in boosting the ability to get to sleep as well as in the quality of the sleep. However, the Halcion® group felt hangover symptoms and had trouble concentrating the next day, while those taking the valerian/lemon balm combination reported no negative effect.[168]

In dealing with sleep disorders it is important to recognise that not all people have the same sleeping requirements. As a person gets to be 50 or 55, he or she usually will require less sleep. Some people can get by quite nicely with 4 to 6 hours' sleep at night and a catnap during the day. The real criterion as to whether a person is getting enough sleep is his or her general health and energy levels. If a person does not sleep until one or two in the morning but feels fine and has plenty of energy, then there is no problem. On the other hand if that person lays awake fretting about not being asleep – then there may be a sleep disorder.

Relaxation techniques are a very good way of helping induce sleep. There are many audio tapes that can be played before going to bed and with training and determination, most insomniacs can alleviate their problem. Hypnosis has also been a remedy for many insomniacs. The usual method is to teach the subject self-hypnosis slowly, allowing him to relax and then sleep. Autogenics too, has helped many people.

RECOMMENDATIONS FOR INSOMNIA

DIET	A general balanced-diet consisting of all the main food groups, carbohydrates, low fat proteins, essential fatty acids and water.
INCREASE	Relaxing herbal teas before bed
DECREASE	Coffee, tea, chocolate, all caffeinated drinks. Depending how serious the problem is do not have caffeine after 6pm – earlier if a serious problem.
SUPERFOODS	Manuka honey taken with warm water and chamomile tea taken early evening.
SUPPLEMENTS	Magnesium and calcium in the early evening. If taking any other vitamins, always take in the mornings. B-complex, for example may keep you awake if taken too late in the day.
HERBALS	Black Cohosh – tonic for central nervous system Valerian and Rhodiola
LIFESTYLE CHANGES	Learn relaxation techniques. Investigate buying some relaxation tapes. Take up meditation and visualisation. Reflexology is a wonderful treatment for insomnia. A herb pillow is also beneficial.

MIGRAINE HEADACHES

Migraines are very painful headaches sometimes involving nausea, vomiting, and changes in vision. They usually begin on only one side of the head and may become worse with exposure to light. The exact cause of migraine headaches is not well understood. However, certain features of this debilitating disease are known, making effective prevention and treatment available to many migraine sufferers. There are three main areas to investigate when faced with a client with migraine headaches. These are allergies and food intolerance, hormonal imbalance, and blood sugar abnormality.

The first thing that comes to my mind when faced with a client who suffers frequent migraine headaches is the likelihood of allergies and food sensitivities. Migraine can be triggered by allergies and may be relieved by identifying and avoiding the problem foods.[129] [130] Uncovering these food allergies with the help of a nutritional therapist is often a useful way to prevent migraine. Some migraine sufferers have an impaired ability to break down tyramine, a substance found in many foods such as aged cheeses, red wine, beef and chicken liver, and sauerkraut, which is known to trigger migraine in some people.[131] People with this defect are thought to be more sensitive than others to the effects of tyramine.[132]

Monosodium Glutamate (MSG), a flavouring agent used in many foods, has been reported to trigger migraine headaches. Ingestion of the artificial sweetener aspartame has also been reported to provoke migraine in a small proportion of people.[133] [134] Foods that contain nitrates and nitrites, such as preserved meats, are commonly reported triggers of migraine headaches. Contrary to the commonly held belief of many doctors, chocolate does not appear to play a significant role in triggering migraine headaches.[135]

If the allergy route is unsuccessful, another prominent area connected to migraine attacks is hormonal influences. Many women have migraine attacks linked to their menstrual cycles. Menstrual migraine headaches are thought to be related to fluctuating levels of oestrogen in the body. Hormonally triggered migraine may get worse early in pregnancy but tend to improve later in pregnancy. Researchers point out that oral contraceptive use can result in worsening, improvement, or no change in a woman's migraine.[136] Other researchers have presented evidence that the oral contraceptive pill or oestrogen replacement therapy can provoke or exacerbate migraine. Since the use of these hormones has been linked with an increased risk of stroke, and a history of migraine with aura is also a risk factor for stroke, women with migraine should probably avoid oral contraceptives and oestrogen replacement therapy.[137] Research has shown that migraine sufferers have lowered levels of magnesium that other people[140] and that pre-menopausal woman that suffer migraine headaches benefit from magnesium supplements.[141] One double-blind study showed that 350mg of magnesium per day decreased premenstrual migraines.[142]

Blood-sugar abnormalities are also known to trigger migraine headaches. Some migraine sufferers have an abnormality of blood-sugar regulation known as reactive hypoglycemia. In these people, improvement in the frequency and severity of migraine has been observed when dietary changes designed to control the blood sugar were implemented.[138] This was observed as early as 1949.[139] To control blood sugar levels, eating little and often is recommended, with each meal containing small amounts of protein, which will slow down the absorption of the sugar.

The most frequently used herb for the long-term treatment and prevention of migraines is feverfew. Feverfew inhibits both hyper-aggregation of platelets and the release of serotonin and some inflammatory mediators.[143] Double blind studies show that continuous use of feverfew leads to a reduction in the severity, duration, and frequency of migraine headaches.[144,145,146]

Yet another cause of migraine headaches is thought to be related to abnormal serotonin function in blood vessels,[149] and 5-hydroxy-tryptophan (5–HTP, which is converted by the body into serotonin) may help correct this abnormality. In several double-blind trials, supplementation with 5–HTP (200–600mg per day) has improved migraine, often producing results comparable to those achieved with anti-migraine drugs.[150]

Other factors associated with migraine headaches are people with reactions to salt, lactose-intolerant individuals, high protein diets and smoking.

RECOMMENDATIONS FOR MIGRAINE HEADACHES

DIET	Low protein diets have been used with some success to reduce migraine attacks.[147] [148]
INCREASE	Complex carbohydrates and low fat protein foods.
DECREASE	All refined foods, salt and dairy foods
SUPERFOODS	Super Sprouts, Medicinal Mushrooms and Alfalfa
SUPPLEMENTS	B-Complex (B2 in particular), Fish Oils, Magnesium
HERBALS	Feverfew, Ginger. Valerian, Rhodiola
LIFESTYLE CHANGES	Identify food allergies or intolerances, and stop smoking.

NERVOUS SYSTEM RULE NO 3

Regular exercise and keeping the blood vessels open and the heart strong are essential to keeping our brain and nervous system healthy.

GENERAL RECOMMENDATIONS FOR
THE NERVOUS SYSTEM

DIET **FOODS TO SUPPORT**	A whole food approach to food where quality is more important than quantity. Plenty of fruits, vegetables, nuts and seeds with adequate essential fatty acids, low-fat protein, and plenty of water.
FOODS TO AVOID	All known anti-nutrients: alcohol, caffeine, chemicals found in paint, paint thinner, cleaning fluids, gasoline, kerosene, and lighter fluid. Also aluminium, lead, cadmium, mercury (from dental fillings). All synthetic hormones and all denatured food. Excessive E numbers, additives, preservatives, rancid food and pesticides.
SUPERFOODS	All antioxidant foods and supplements. Carotenoids, flavonoids, vitamins C and E, beta carotene, selenium and antioxidant herbs.
SUPPLEMENTS	B12, Folic Acid, Multivitamin and minerals. Antioxidants A,C,E and selenium, Vitamin E in particular has been shown to directly protect the nerves from oxidative damage and improved neurological function after supplementation.[293]
HERBAL REMEDIES	A herbal formula that not only strengthens the nervous system but benefits the peripheral blood circulation. It helps relieve anxiety and tense muscles. It will gradually build a strong nervous system, which protects the immune system. Valerian is rich in calcium and the passionflower is beneficial for the eyes. The formula includes: Black cohosh, Valerian, Capsicum, Passionflower, Skullcap, Hops and Wood Betony.
LIFESTYLE CHANGES	Exercise your brain by exercising your body and avoid free radicals at all costs.

THE REPRODUCTIVE SYSTEM

What is the Reproductive system?

It is the system of the body, which enables reproduction to take place thereby maintaining the species. The reproductive systems differ in males and females.

Main function:

Maintains the continuation of the human species.

What does the Reproductive system actually do?

Reproduction is the process by which genetic material is passed from generation to generation. In this regard reproduction maintains the continuation of the species. Reproduction is also the process by which a single cell duplicates its genetic material allowing an organism to grow and repair itself, thus, reproduction maintains the life of the individual.

The organs of the reproductive system are grouped as gonads, ducts and accessory sex glands. The male structures of reproduction include the testes, ductus epididymis, vas deferens, ejaculatory duct, urethra, seminal vesicles, prostate gland, Cowper's glands and penis. The female structures of reproduction include the ovaries, Fallopian tubes, uterus, vagina and vulva. The mammary glands are also considered part of the reproductive system.

The coming together of a male and a female in the act of unprotected sexual intercourse is the process by which spermatozoa provided by the male are deposited in the vagina of the female. The end result of which could be pregnancy. Pregnancy is a sequence of events that normally includes fertilisation, implantation, embryonic growth and fetal growth that terminates in birth.

Dietary influences affecting the reproductive system

The sperm count in males has decreased 50% over the last 50 years and whereas our grandmothers and mothers were likely to get pregnant with their first encounter with sexual intercourse, now one in four couples have difficulty in conceiving even after one year of trying. These are quite an amazing statistics – and one of the main reasons behind them is poor diet. Latest research has shown that our fruit and vegetables have at least 50 per cent less minerals and vitamins than in the fruit and vegetables of 50 years ago. That, together with our modern fast lifestyles, fast adulterated food, alcohol and stress have all had their part to play in affecting the reproductive system. More than any other system of the body, the reproductive system needs fresh, unadulterated foods of the richest and most natural quality. To function optimally, the reproductive system needs the B complex of vitamins, complete proteins, marine oils, vitamins A, C, E and the minerals selenium and zinc – all of which are depleted in many people.

REPRODUCTIVE SYSTEM RULE NO 1

More than any other system of the body, the reproductive system needs fresh, unadulterated foods of the richest and most natural quality.

COMMON DISORDERS
INFERTILITY

Infertility in its strictest definition means 'failure to reproduce' after an unprotected intercourse. Many doctors suggest that if a couple has been trying to conceive a baby for 18 months without success, and having regular unprotected sex two or three times a week they should go to their GP and ask to be referred to a specialist unit to find out why. Some specialists suggest you take action sooner than that. Couples over 30 should wait only a year before seeking advice and for women over 36 should wait no longer than six months. Female fertility peaks between 24 and 27 then declines slowly but surely thereafter.

20% of couples conceive within one month of trying and about 50% of fertile couples will conceive within 6 months of trying with 85% being successful within one year. The remaining 15% may have a fertility problem.

Female Infertility

There are many reasons for not conceiving. It can be caused by sex-hormone abnormalities, low thyroid function, endometriosis, scarring of the Fallopian tubes, or a host of other causes. Some of the causes of infertility readily respond to natural medicine whereas others do not. There are many dietary and nutritional changes that may be helpful. Caffeine consumption equivalent to more than three cups of coffee per day has been linked to tubal disease and endometriosis – both of which can cause female infertility.[208] As little as one to one and a half cups of coffee per day appears to delay conception in women trying to get pregnant.[209] Some studies find one cup of coffee per day cuts fertility in half[209] although others report that it takes two, or three to have detrimental effects. Caffeine is found in regular coffee, black and green tea, some soft drinks, chocolate and many over the counter pharmaceuticals. While not every study finds that caffeine reduces female fertility, most nutritional therapists recommend that women trying to get pregnant avoid caffeine altogether.

Excessive or insufficient weight, smoking and even moderate amounts of alcohol are also likely to reduce the chance of conceiving. The more women smoke, the less likely the chance to conceive.[210] In fact, women whose mothers smoked during *their* pregnancy are only half as likely to conceive as those whose mothers were non-smokers.[211]

Studies have shown that being deficient in iron and the B vitamins reduce female fertility, whereas a double blind research trial has shown that taking a multivitamin/mineral supplement increases female fertility.[212] Studies have shown that vitamin E deficiency in animals leads to infertility and a preliminary trial on humans, when 100ius of vitamin E were given to both men and women of infertile couples resulted in a significant increase in fertility.[213]

The Pill – if a women has been taking the Pill for a few years and then stops and switches to another form of contraception, her cycles can be erratic for up to 4 or 5 months. There is anecdotal evidence that a small number of women may find conception difficult after a long period of Pill taking.

IDU's can increase the chances of pelvic infection threefold. This can affect fertility if the infection reaches the Fallopian tubes and is severe enough to block them with scar tissue.

Smoking – this can affect a woman's (and a man's) fertility by causing constriction of the blood vessels including those supporting the reproductive organs, thus inhibiting their proper function. It can also act directly on the tiny cilia lining the Fallopian tubes inhibiting their action too.

Endometriosis – pieces of womb lining can migrate to other places in the pelvis such as the Fallopian tubes or around the ovaries. Like the rest of the womb lining they are still under the control of your hormones, so they continue to shed blood each month wherever they are. This can occasionally block the tubes or more often, clog the area around the ovaries so the ripened egg cannot get out.

Ovulation problems – ovulation problems occur if the ovaries are damaged, not working in a cycle or the cause is hormonal or chemical.

Male Infertility

The two most important nutrients to improve male fertility are vitamin C and zinc. Vitamin C protects sperm from oxidative damage[214] and improves the quality of sperm in smokers. Where sperm stick together (a condition called agglutination), fertility is reduced. Vitamin C reduces sperm agglutination,[215] increasing the fertility of men with this condition. A minimum 1g of vitamin C daily is recommended.

A lack of zinc can reduce testosterone levels.[216] For men with low testosterone levels, supplementation raises testosterone and also increases fertility.[217] For men with low serum zinc levels, zinc supplements may increase both sperm counts and fertility.[218] Most studies have infertile men take zinc supplements for at least several months. The ideal amount of supplemental zinc remains unknown but I usually recommend 30mg of zinc taken daily in the evenings. Liquid zinc can be purchased and is said to be absorbed more efficiently. Minerals, including zinc, should be taken in evenings when they are better absorbed.

Co-Q-10 is a nutrient used by the body in the production of energy. While its energy role in the formation of sperm is unknown, there is evidence that as little as 10mg per day (over a two-week period) will increase sperm count and motility.[219]

RECOMMENDATIONS FOR FEMALE INFERTILITY

DIET	A whole food approach. Nothing denatured, or from packets containing additives. Fresh good quality, preferably organic foods.
INCREASE	Everything healthy – green leafy vegetables, fruit, lean meat and poultry. Lots of water.
DECREASE	Coffee, alcohol, and all refined foods.
SUPERFOODS	Oysters, asparagus, algae, Manuka honey
SUPPLEMENTS	Pregnancy Pack – *or* A Multivitamin/Mineral with added 20mg zinc. Fish Oils Folic Acid
HERBALS	Vitex
LIFESTYLE CHANGES	Avoid all caffeinated substances. Rule out iron deficiency. Relax

REPRODUCTIVE SYSTEM RULE NO 2

Zinc supplementation should always be considered for men and women experiencing infertility problems.

RECOMMENDATIONS FOR MALE INFERTILITY

DIET	A whole food approach. Nothing denatured, or from packets containing additives. Fresh good quality, preferably organic foods.
INCREASE	Everything healthy – green leafy vegetables, fruit, lean meat and poultry. Lots of water
DECREASE	Coffee. Alcohol, all refined foods.
SUPERFOODS	Oysters, asparagus, algae, Manuka honey
SUPPLEMENTS	A Multivitamin/Mineral 25mg zinc. 1g vitamin C daily. Fish Oils
HERBALS	Vitex
LIFESTYLE CHANGES	Avoid all caffeinated substances. Rule out zinc deficiency. Relax

THE FEMALE CYCLE

The average menstrual cycle lasts for 28 days although it is not uncommon for cycles to vary between three to six weeks. Emotional states, stress, diet, other hormones, illness and drugs can all affect menstruation. The majority of women have knowledge of the roles of oestrogen and progesterone in their bodies, but few are aware of the other two very important hormones that have just as important roles. These are Follicle Stimulating hormone (FS) and the Luteinizing hormone (LH).

Days 1–14 of the menstrual cycle are the days from menstruation to ovulation. At the beginning of the cycle the levels of hormones oestrogen and progesterone are very low as a result of the shedding of the womb lining. The hypothalamus in the brain is the master gland of this hormonal activity and when it senses that the levels are low it releases the first master hormone which causes the pituitary gland to release follicle stimulating hormone (FSH). It is this hormone that ripens one egg within the ovary for release into the Fallopian tube. FSH also stimulates the production of estrogen by the ovary, which increases over the first fourteen days of the cycle, bringing about the growth of the lining of the womb and breast tissue.

When oestrogen levels peak around day 12 of the cycle, the hypothalamus gland then releases luteinizing hormone (LH). On day 14 of a normal cycle, a surge of luteinizing hormone brings about ovulation, the release of a mature egg from one of the ovaries. This egg then travels through the Fallopian tube towards the uterus.

Days 14–28 of the menstrual cycle are the days from ovulation to menstruation. During this second half of the cycle there are high levels of both oestrogen and progesterone to support fertilisation should it occur. Progesterone starts its increase just after ovulation and increases body temperature by at least 0.2 centigrade. Many women therefore take their temperature in order to check whether they have ovulated. If the egg is not fertilised, the lining of the womb is released forming the menstrual flow. This causes a rapid fall in the levels of oestrogens and progesterone, and the low levels act as a signal for the hypothalamus gland to release its master hormone and the process starts all over again.

Luteinizing hormones and follicle stimulating hormones are important indicators in cases of infertility, PMS, and menopause. You can now be tested over a one-month period for all four of the main hormones to monitor their progress throughout the month. This is carried out by a 28 day saliva test and the results are often most interesting. Whilst these tests can be of immense value, they are also expensive and it must be remembered that emotional states, stress, diet, other hormones, illness and drugs can all affect menstruation, and therefore maybe the test results too.

DYSMENORRHEOA (HEAVY PERIODS)

Dysmenorrheoa, or painful menstruation, is classified as either primary or secondary. Primary dysmenorrheoa generally occurs within a couple of years of the first menstruation period. The pain tends to decrease with age and very often resolves after childbirth. Secondary dysmenorrheoa is commonly a result of endometriosis, starts later in life, and tends to increase in intensity over time. As many as half of menstruating women are affected by dysmenorrhoea, and of these 10 per cent have severe dysmenorrhoea, which greatly limits activities for one to three days every month.[219]

Women suffering from this miserable monthly experience have their own solutions to menstrual cramps. Some women find gentle exercise helpful while others do not; and some feel the need just to lie still. There are however, several lifestyle changes and nutritional supplements that may be helpful.

Many studies have reported that alcohol should be avoided by women experiencing menstrual pain, because it depletes stores of certain nutrients and alters the metabolism of carbohydrates — which in turn worsen muscle spasms. Alcohol can also interfere with the liver's ability to metabolise hormones. In theory, this might result in elevated oestrogen levels, increased fluid retention and heavier menstrual flow.

Niacin has been reported to be effective in relieving menstrual cramps. In one study, 87 per cent of a group of forty women reported benefit from the supplement. In theory, calcium may help prevent menstrual cramp, as muscles that are calcium-deficient tend to be hyperactive and therefore might be more prone to cramp. Whilst calcium could be beneficial for cramping, it is advisable to always supplement calcium with magnesium.

In one double blind trial, fish oil led to a statistically significant 37 per cent drop in menstrual symptoms. In that report, adolescent girls with dysmenorrhoea were given 1,080mg of EPA and 720mg of DHA per day for two months to achieve this result.[220] This would amount to 6,000mg fish oil per day. The Danish have carried out many studies using fish oil alone, fish oil with vitamin B12 and vitamin B12 alone, and have found that women who suffer painful periods appear to be deficient in both nutrients. By including fatty fish in the diet three times per week, could ease their monthly cramps. Oily fish are sardines, tuna, salmon, herring and mackerel. The amounts of B12 used were small at just 7.5mcg daily. However, because of the different types of dysmenorrhoea, it would be wise to seek advice from a nutritional therapist before selecting supplements. If the underlying cause were endometriosis, this would have to be taken into account.

Black cohosh has a history as a folk medicine for relieving menstrual cramps. Black cohosh can be taken in several forms, including crude, dried root, or rhizome (300–2,000mg per day) or as a solid, dry powdered extract (250mg three times per day). Standardized extracts of the herb are probably the easiest to take. Dong Quai is a traditional Chinese herb that may also ease dysmenorrhoea. The powdered root can be used or in capsules, tablets, tinctures or as a tea. This herb is known as an 'adaptogen' and has the ability to normalise female hormones.

The Contraceptive Pill. A review of literature suggests that women who use oral contraceptives may experience decreased vitamin B1, B2, B3, B12, C and zinc levels. Synthetic hormones disrupt the endocrine system so you may wish to investigate alternative methods of birth control.

AMENORRHOEA – LACK OF PERIODS

Amenorrhoea is usually associated with strict dieting and/or strenuous exercise although there can be other causes. Our bodies are composed of a mixture of fat, a fat-free mass or lean tissue, and a glycogen store. It is normal and indeed necessary for everyone to have a certain amount of fat in their bodies.. A woman needs to have at least 22 per cent of her body weight as fat in order to have regular periods. Many women with anorexia nervosa or are underweight do not have periods for this reason. However, having regular periods also relies on hormones. Hormones can be affected by dieting and weight loss, so even when she has enough body fat, a woman's period may become irregular or stop.

The reproductive system heavily relies on zinc, and this supplement would be the first choice for aiming to rebalance the body and to start menstruation again. Liquid zinc would be recommended for better absorption. This is a serious problem and should not be overlooked. A nutritional therapist will be able to offer much advice with *disordered eating* leading to too much weight loss, but in some cases a referral to a specially trained counsellor in *eating disorders* may be necessary. In any event a visit to the GP should be the first port of call.

IRREGULAR PERIODS

Irregular periods may be perfectly normal, especially as women reach the menopause years, where they will probably become irregular before stopping altogether. Irregular periods are associated with extreme stress, the contraceptive pill, strenuous exercise, low weight and anorexia nervosa. If you're periods are not regular and you are not menopause age then it may be worth checking it out. In the meantime, a whole food approach to food taking in all the main food groups with each meal will be a good start.

RECOMMENDATIONS FOR HEAVY PERIODS

DIET	A whole food approach to food. Good nourishing food with plenty of fruits and vegetables, low fat protein, and plenty of water.
INCREASE	Fatty fish, fruit and vegetables
DECREASE	Alcohol, red meat, refined foods, chocolate,
SUPERFOODS	Yoghurt, Alfalfa, Honey, Bee Pollen, Barley Grass
SUPPLEMENTS	A good multivitamin/mineral. B6 and zinc taken for the second half of the cycle has been said to be beneficial. Zinc and vitamin C and bioflavonoids
HERBALS	Black cohosh, Valerian
LIFESTYLE CHANGES	Test for food intolerance. Taking vitamin C with iron rich foods increases the absorption of iron.

REPRODUCTIVE SYSTEM RULE NO 3
For a healthy reproductive system,
AVOID alcohol, saturated fats and sugar

ENDOMETRIOSIS

The endometrium is the lining of the uterus (womb). Every month hormones in the blood prepare it to support and nourish a fertilised egg. If there is no pregnancy, the endometrium is shed during your period. It comes out through your cervix (neck of womb) but some also travels back up through the Fallopian tubes and spills into your abdominal cavity. This is quite normal and usually causes no problems. The stray endometrial cells are simply absorbed. With endometriosis however, some of these cells implant and start to grow. The result can be pain, scarring and infertility – although how this happens is not fully understood. The main symptoms are infertility, painful periods (dysmenorrhoea), painful sex (dyspareunia), painful bowel movements or painful urination. Other symptoms include painful ovulation, a swollen abdomen, a loss of old brown blood and blood clots during periods, irregular periods and, not surprisingly depression and other psychological problems.

Endometriosis is therefore a condition where cells that are normally located **inside** the uterus are found **outside** the uterus, most often in the pelvic cavity. Endometriosis lesions have been found on nearly every organ in the female body, but are most frequently located on the reproductive organs, the bladder, bowel, intestines, colon and appendix. When active, endometriosis lesions respond to a woman's hormones each month. As a result the lesions can inflame surrounding tissue and cause bleeding and scarring. It is estimated that 30–40 per cent of women with endometriosis are also infertile.

The precise cause of endometriosis is not known but there are plenty of theories. Misplaced endometrial cells meant for the lining of the womb which were formed before birth and ended up in the wrong place, is one theory. Retrograde menstruation (bleeding upwards into the Fallopian tubes) instead of downwards and out through the vagina is the other main theory. 90% of women have some degree of retrograde menstruation and they don't all get endometriosis but for those that do it is thought are unable to clear it from the abdominal cavity.

Another possible cause is the link between dioxin exposure and the development of endometriosis. In one study on rhesus monkeys, 79 per cent of the monkeys exposed to dioxin developed endometriosis. Further, the monkeys who had the most exposure had the most extensive endometriosis. Dioxins are part of the organochlorine group of chemicals. Studies have shown that organochlorines act as hormones in our bodies. Dioxin is created by incinerators burning chlorinated waste, leaded gas and in the manufacture of pesticides, solvents and PVC plastics. Dioxin can be found in bleached products, and most alarmingly may be found in women's sanitary products except those manufactured specifically without dioxins.

When endometriosis affects reproductive organs such as when adhesions block the Fallopian tubes or when an endometrioma on the ovary prevents ovulation, then fertility is compromised. Loss of fertility is investigated in at least half of those with endometriosis as 30 to 40 per cent of sufferers cannot conceive.

There is no quick and simple test to diagnose endometriosis. Only a doctor can do this by examination and the best time for this is just before a period. After ruling out other possible problems which could be causing symptoms such as PID (pelvic inflammatory disease) or various bowel or bladder disorders, the doctor may recommend a laparoscopy. (surgery in which a light is inserted into small incisions in the abdomen).

Dietary advice for endometriosis - because of the precise cause of endometriosis has never been established treatment is not certain. There is much evidence that excessive candida in the system creates blockages in the Fallopian tubes, thereby causing a leak of cells into the endometrium. If you think candida is at the root of the problem, recommend the anti-candida diet regime. Therapists using this treatment with endometriosis clients have achieved good results.

RECOMMENDATIONS FOR ENDOMETRIOSIS

DIET	A whole food approach to food where quality is more important than quantity. Plenty of fruits and vegetables, low-fat protein, and plenty of water.
INCREASE	Whole grains, oily fish, fresh fruit and vegetables, preferably organic.
DECREASE	Avoid all pesticides, all junk food, everything refined, especially chocolate, white rice and bread.
SUPERFOODS	Bee Pollen, Medicinal Mushrooms, Barley Grass, Algae
SUPPLEMENTS	A good multivitamin/mineral containing no less than 50mg of all the B-complex vitamins. Antioxidants
HERBALS	Don Quai, Black cohosh, Ginkgo Biloba
LIFESTYLE CHANGES	Avoid all synthetic hormones. Avoid tampons, or buy sanitary wear specially prepared without bleach.

IMPOTENCE

Impotence, or erectile dysfunction, is the inability of a male to attain or sustain an erection sufficient for intercourse. It can be a persistent condition; however, almost half of all men experience impotence occasionally. Impotence can have either physical or psychological (or both) causes. Although some doctors used to believe differently, most researchers and doctors now believe that a majority of men suffering from impotence have physical causes. Psychological counselling can be helpful if the impotence is related to emotional factors. There are several physical contributors to impotence, including atherosclerosis, diabetes, hypothyroidism, multiple sclerosis, and chronic alcohol use.

Impotence that cannot be linked to physical causes has been successfully treated by hypnosis.[118] In this trial, three hypnosis sessions per week were used initially, later decreasing to one per month during a six-month period. Three out of every four men in the trial were helped.

Dilation of blood vessels necessary for a normal erection depends on a substance called nitric oxide. In turn, the amino acid arginine is needed for nitric oxide formation. In a group of fifteen men with erectile dysfunction given 2,800mg arginine per day for two weeks, six were helped, though none improved while taking placebo.[119]

Low blood levels of the hormone DHEA have been reported in some men with erectile dysfunction. In one double blind trial, forty men with low DHEA levels and impotence were given 50mg of DHEA for six months.[221] Significant improvement in both erectile function and interest in sex occurred in the men assigned DHEA but not in those assigned to placebo. No significant change occurred in testosterone levels or in factors that could affect the prostate gland. Experts have concerns about the safe use of DHEA, particularly because long-term safety data do not exist.

There are a number of herbs that may be helpful for impotence. Damiana and Asian ginseng are traditional herbs for impotent men, however no modern studies have confirmed their effectiveness. Ginkgo Biloba, which is a herb often recommended for circulatory problems, may help some impotent men[222] by increasing arterial blood flow.

The herb that offers the most promising results however, is Yohimbe. Yohimbe dilates blood vessels, making this herb useful for treating male impotence. Yohimbine (the primary active constituent in yohimbe) has been shown in several double blind studies to help treatment with impotence.[223] [224] Somewhat surprisingly, yohimbe appears to help regardless of the cause of impotence. A tincture of yohimbe bark is often used in the amount of 5–6 drops three times per day. There are also standardized yohimbe products available. A typical daily amount of yohimbine is 15–30mg, however, it is best to take this herb under the supervision of a nutritional therapist with experience of herbal remedies.

RECOMMENDATIONS FOR IMPOTENCE

DIET	A whole food approach to food. Good nourishing food with plenty of fruits and vegetables, low-fat protein, and plenty of water.
INCREASE	All fruits and vegetables
DECREASE	All refined foods, alcohol, cigarettes
SUPERFOODS	Bee Pollen, Honey, Medicinal mushrooms, super sprouts
SUPPLEMENTS	A good multivitamin/mineral DHEA, arginine, zinc, folic acid
HERBALS	Yohimbe, Gingko Biloba -
LIFESTYLE CHANGES	Learn relaxation techniques. Look into hypnosis. Take up yoga and reduce stress levels.

PRE MENSTRUAL SYNDROME

The symptoms of PMS are wide ranging and include cramping, bloating, mood swings, breast tenderness, irritability, fatigue, head-aches and depression. Premenstrual symptoms typically begin at the end of each monthly cycle and resolve with the start of menstruation.

Women who eat more sugary foods appear to have an increased risk of PMS.[225] Alcohol can affect hormone metabolism and women who drink heavily are more likely to suffer with symptoms than non drinking women. In one study of Chinese women, increasing tea consumption was associated with increasing prevalence of PMS and among a group of college students in the United States, consummation of caffeine-containing beverages was associated with increases in both the prevalence and severity of PMS.[226] Moreover, the more caffeine women consumed, the more likely the chance to suffer from symp-toms.[227] Therefore, nutritional recommendations based on the scient-ific studies would be to avoid sugar, alcohol and caffeine, especially during the second half of your monthly cycle. Several other studies have shown that diets low in fat or high in fiber may help to reduce symptoms of PMS.

Exercise is helpful and often recommended to reduce PMS symptoms. Women with PMS who jogged an average of about twelve miles a week for six months experienced a reduction in breast tenderness, fluid retention, depression and stress.[228]

Many nutritional supplements help relieve PMS symptoms and the most successful is Vitamin B6 and zinc. It is recommended that a specifically blended supplement be bought containing B6 and zinc and taken for the last two weeks of the cycle.

According to studies, many women with PMS have been shown unable to convert linoleic acid to gamma linolenic acid (GLA). Many things including stress, poor diet, alcohol, and a lack of certain nutrients impair conversion. Supplementation of Evening Primrose oil therefore, which contains significant amounts of GLA, can bypass this conversion by putting GLA directly into the body. Starflower oil also contains GLA in higher quantities, but some research has shown that the GLA from Evening Primrose oil is better absorbed. Whilst addressing many of the PMS symptoms, EPO (Evening Primrose Oil) specifically helped women who experience breast tenderness or fibrocystic breast disease.[229]

Other nutrients that are beneficial are calcium, magnesium, and vitamin E. One study on vitamin E showed that whilst many women are not vitamin E deficient, a small supplement of 300ius daily, decreased PMS symptoms.

Herbal remedies that can be helpful are Don Quai, Black Cohosh, Vitex. Don Quai is often referred to as a 'female ginseng'. It is an adaptogenic herb that helps promote normal hormone balance and is particularly useful for women experiencing premenstrual cramping and pain.

Vitex has been shown to help re-establish normal balance of oestrogen and progesterone during a woman's menstrual cycle. This is important

because some women suffer from PMS and other menstrual irregularities due to underproduction of the hormone progesterone during the
second half of their cycle. Vitex stimulates the pituitary gland to
produce more luteinizing hormone, and this leads to greater productivity of progesterone.[230] Studies have shown that using Vitex once in the
morning over a period of several months helps normalise hormone
balance to alleviate the symptoms of PMS. One study showed Vitex to
be as effective as 200mg of vitamin B6 in a double blind study.[231]

RECOMMENDATIONS FOR PMS

DIET	Low in meat and dairy and high in fruit, vegetables and whole grains.
INCREASE	Water, fruit and vegetables, good quality, low-fat protein
DECREASE	Red meat, avoid sugar, alcohol and caffeine
SUPERFOODS	Alfalfa, Algae, Barley Grass, Medicinal mushrooms and yoghurt.
SUPPLEMENTS	A good multivitamin/mineral. Calcium:Magnesium
HERBALS	Don Quai, Vitex or Black Cohosh. (or a combination of all three)
LIFESTYLE CHANGES	Regular exercise has been proved to be beneficial in fluid retention, breast tenderness, depression and stress

GENERAL RECOMMENDATIONS FOR THE REPRODUCTIVE SYSTEM

DIET **FOODS TO SUPPORT**	More than any other system of the body, the reproductive system needs fresh, unadulterated foods of the richest and most natural quality. Good sources of folic acid are Brussel sprouts, Marmite, cornflakes, baked beans, lettuce and broccoli.
FOODS TO AVOID	All junk food – that includes all refined foods, anything with additives or pesticides, all ready-made meals, alcohol, saturated fat and sugars of all kinds.
SUPERFOODS	Alfalfa, Algae, Barley Grass, Medicinal mushrooms, yoghurt. Bee Pollen, Honey, Super sprouts
SUPPLEMENTS	A good multivitamin/mineral would be the base of a supplement programme for the reproductive system as a whole. Additional folic acid for women would be recommended if trying to become pregnant and additional zinc for both male and females also if trying to conceive. Pregnancy Pack is a good supplement for before, during and after pregnancy. Fish Oils are highly recommended. Combination supplements of EPA/DHA are available.
HERBAL REMEDIES	Don Quai, Vitex, Black Cohosh (or a combination). Valerian and/or Ginkgo Biloba.
LIFESTYLE CHANGES	Test for food intolerance/allergy. Taking vitamin C with iron rich foods increases the absorption of iron. (a boiled egg and a glass of orange juice for example). Regular exercise has been proved to be beneficial in fluid retention, breast tenderness, depression and stress. Learn relaxation techniques. Look into hypnosis. Take up yoga and reduce stress levels.

THE RESPIRATORY SYSTEM

What is the Respiratory system?

The respiratory system is the system in the body responsible for the exchange of gases in the lungs.

Main function:

To continuously supply oxygen to every cell in the body for various metabolic reactions and to remove carbon dioxide, a waste product of those cells, that need to be eliminated quickly from the body.

What does the Respiratory system actually do?

The respiratory system consists of the nose, naso-pharynx, pharynx, larynx, trachea, bronchi and the lungs, which provide the passageway for air in and out of the body.

Oxygen is taken in through the nose and mouth and flows along the trachea and bronchial tubes to the alveoli of the lungs, where it diffused through the thin film of moisture lining the alveoli. The inspired air, which is now rich with oxygen, comes into contact with the blood in the capillary network surrounding the alveoli. The oxygen then diffuses across a permeable membrane wall surrounding the alveoli to be taken up by red blood cells and carried to the heart. Carbon dioxide, collected by the respiring cells around the body, passes in the opposite direction by diffusing from the capillary walls into the alveoli, to be passed through the bronchi and trachea and exhaled through the nose and mouth.

Dietary influences affecting the respiratory system

Foods that we have used for centuries to fight respiratory diseases are very similar to the drugs we use today. They have a common action in that they thin out and help move the lung's secretions so that they do not clog air passages and can be coughed up or normally expelled. Such foods and drugs are called 'mucokinetic' (mucus moving) agents, and include decongestants and expectorants. Many clients who suffer with respiratory problems also have a diet high in acid forming foods (meat, cheese, eggs). Excess milk and dairy products therefore are the group of foods most likely to affect the respiratory system in a negative way in that they are acid and mucus forming.

Chilli peppers and hot pungent foods on the other hand, are top of the list for assisting respiratory diseases. The mouth-burning ingredient in hot red peppers is capsaicin, which has some chemical resemblance to the drug Guaifenesin. Guaifenesin in an expectorant, found in about 75% of OTC (over the counter) and prescription cough syrups, cold tablets and expectorants such as Vicks Formula 440, Sudafed and Robitussin.

Allicin, which gives garlic its flavour, is converted in the body to a drug similar to S-carboxymethyl-cystein (Mucodyne), a classic European lung medication that regulates mucus flow.

> 'A lot of over the counter drugs for colds, coughs and bronchitis do exactly what peppers do, but I believe more in peppers. Peppers don't cause any side effects. I am convinced that 90% of all people can tolerate hot food and get a benefit'.
> **Dr. Irwin Ziment – Lung Specialist at UCLA**

COMMON DISORDERS
ASTHMA

Asthma is a lung disorder in which spasms of the bronchial passages restrict the flow in and out of the lungs. Asthma may be described as an allergic reaction that occurs in the airways of the lungs. In asthma white cells in the bronchi secrete histamine, making the smooth muscle cells of the lung airways contract more readily. The number of people with asthma and the death rate from this condition have been increasing since the late 1980s, and some suggest that environmental pollution may be the causes of this growing epidemic.

Some asthmatics react to food additives such as sulfites, tartrazine (yellow dye) and aspirin-like substances found in foods called natural salicylates.[232] [233] Although most people with asthma do not suffer from food allergies, unrecognised food allergy can be an exacerbating factor.[234]

Vitamin B6 deficiency is common in asthmatics. This deficiency may relate to the asthma itself or to certain asthma drugs that deplete vitamin B6.[234] In a double blind study of asthmatic children, 200mg per day of vitamin B6 for two months reduced the severity of their illness and reduced the amount of asthma medication needed. In another study asthmatic adults experienced a dramatic decrease in the frequency and severity of asthma attacks while taking 50mg of vitamin B6 twice a day.[236]

Studies have shown that magnesium levels are frequently low in asthmatics. Magnesium may prevent asthma attacks because magnesium can prevent spasms of the bronchial passages. Intravenous injection of magnesium has been reported to stop acute asthma attacks within minutes in double blind research. Although the effect of oral magnesium has not been appropriately studied, many nutritional therapists recommend magnesium supplementation to their asthma clients. The usual amount would be 200–400mg per day.

Supplementation with 1 gram of vitamin C per day reduces the tendency of the bronchial passages to go into spasm,[237] an action that has been confirmed in double blind research. Some individuals with asthma have shown improvement after taking 1–2 grams of vitamin C per day. A buffered form of vitamin C (such as sodium ascorbate or calcium ascorbate) work better for some asthmatics than regular vitamin C (ascorbic acid).[238]

People with low levels of selenium have a high risk of asthma, according to many studies. Asthma involves free radical damage that selenium might protect against. A double blind trial gave 45mcg of selenium to twelve people with asthma. Half showed clear clinical improvement even though lung function tests did not change. Many nutritional therapists recommend 200mcg per day of selenium for adults with asthma, and a proportionately reduced amount for children.

Double blind research shows that fish oil partially reduces reactions to allergens that can trigger attacks in some asthmatics, and further research suggests that children who eat oily fish may have a much lower risk of getting asthma. Therefore, even though evidence supporting the use of fish oils remains weak, eating fish may still be worth considering.

Quercetin, a flavonoid found in most plants, has an inhibiting action on lipoxygenase, an enzyme that contributes to problems with asthma,[239] and whilst no human studies have confirmed whether Quercetin decreases asthma symptoms, many nutritional therapists use this supplement with beneficial results.

Traditionally, herbs that have a soothing action on bronchioles are also used for asthma. These would include marshmallow and liquorice.

Bromelain reduces the thickness of mucus, which may be beneficial for those with asthma, though clinical actions in asthmatics remain unproved.

RECOMMENDATIONS FOR ASTHMA

DIET	A low dairy diet recommended.
INCREASE	Fresh green leafy vegetables, and fruit – preferably organic, and always well washed.
DECREASE	Caffeine, sugar, salt and chlorinated tap water.
SUPERFOODS	Algae, Alfalfa, Cabbage, Honey, Super Sprouts, Manuka Honey, Liquorice.
SUPPLEMENTS	Selenium and Vitamin B6.
HERBALS	Liquorice, Ginkgo Biloba and Marshmallow.
LIFESTYLE CHANGES	Have possible allergens identified. Reduce stress as much as possible and practice yoga techniques.

RESPIRATORY SYSTEM RULE NO 1

ANY FOOD – NO MATTER HOW HEALTHY MAY INDUCE AN ALLERGIC REACTION – REMAIN AWARE OF WHAT YOU ARE EATING AND WHEN

BRONCHITIS

Bronchitis is an inflammation of the trachea and bronchial tree and can be either acute or chronic. Acute bronchitis may be caused by viral or bacterial infections and is preceded by an upper respiratory tract infection. In addition, acute bronchitis can result in irritation of the mucous membranes by environmental fumes, acids, solvents, or tobacco smoke. While smoking is a very health damaging practice and not recommended, studies have now shown that eating fish can decrease some of the damage to the lungs, even in adults who smoke. Comparing smokers who ate fish four times a week with those who ate fish less than once a week, one study showed that the high fish consumers cut their incidence of chronic bronchitis and emphysema by an incredible 45 per cent.

Bronchitis usually begins with a dry, non-productive cough. After a few hours or days, the cough may become more frequent and produce mucus. A secondary bacterial infection may occur, in which the sputum (bronchial secretions) may contain pus. If symptoms persist then a visit to the GP will be necessary.

Dietary factors may influence both inflammatory activity and antioxidant status in the body. Increased inflammation and decreased antioxidant activity each may lead to an increased incidence of chronic diseases, such as chronic bronchitis. People suffering from chronic bronchitis may experience an improvement in symptoms when consuming a diet high in anti-inflammatory fatty acids, such as those found in fish.

A diet high in antioxidants may protect against the free radical damaging effect of the toxins. Studies comparing different populations have shown that increasing fruit and vegetable consumption may reduce the risk of developing chronic bronchitis.

Food and environmental allergies may be triggering factors in some cases of chronic bronchitis.[255] Many nutritional therapists believe that dairy products can increase mucus production, and that people suffering from either acute or chronic bronchitis should therefore limit their intake of dairy products. Ingestion of simple sugars such as sucrose and fructose can lead to suppression of immune function[256] therefore sugars should be avoided in the diet.

In a study of elderly patients hospitalised with acute bronchitis, those who were given 200mg per day of vitamin C improved to significantly greater extent, compared with those who were given a placebo.[257]

Vitamin A status is low in children with measles, an infection that can result in pneumonia or other respiratory complications. Supplementation with vitamin A has been found to decrease morbidity and mortality from measles. In another study supplementation with vitamin A reduced the number of respiratory tract infections in children.

In a double blind study, individuals with chronic bronchitis who received N-acetyl cycsteine (NAC; 600mg a day, three days a week by mouth) had a significant reduction in the number of exacerbations of their illness.[258] Smokers have also been found to benefit from taking NAC.[259] In addition to helping break up mucus, NAC may reduce the elevated bacterial counts that are often seen in the lungs of smokers with chronic bronchitis.[260]

The thymus gland plays a number of important roles in the functioning of the immune system. An extract from calf thymus gland known as thymomudulin has been found in double blind study, to decrease the frequency of respiratory infections in children who are prone to such infections.

The herbs that are beneficial for the respiratory system and for bronchitis in particular are liquorice, thyme, echinacea, and garlic.

Liquorice acts as an anti-inflammatory and antitussive agent. Thyme contains an essential oil (thymol) and certain flavonoids. This plant has anti-spasmodic and expectorant properties and antibacterial actions, and it is considered in cases of bronchitis.[261]

Echinacea is widely used by herbalists for individuals with acute respiratory infection. This herb stimulates the immune system in different ways such as enhancing macrophage function and increasing T-cell response. Echinacea also contains an antibiotic compound known as echinacoside. This herb may therefore be useful for preventing a cold, flu or viral bronchitis from progressing to a secondary bacterial infection.

Garlic has been shown to have mild antimicrobial activity and therefore may be of value with people with bronchitis.

RECOMMENDATIONS FOR BRONCHITIS

DIET	An alkaline diet is recommended for as long as symptoms persist. Citrus juice and fruit, Green vegetable juice plus raw salads, and onions – cooked and raw.
INCREASE	Hot water, lemon and Manuka honey, Herbal teas, garlic.
DECREASE	Everything refined – especially white bread and flour, confectionery, and alcohol.
SUPERFOODS	Liquorice, Alfalfa, Chlorella, Barley Grass, Bee Pollen, Cabbage, Manuka Honey (in hot drinks). Medicinal mushrooms, Super Sprouts.
SUPPLEMENTS	N-acetyl cysteine (NAC), Thymus glandular. Vitamins C, and E. Vitamin A is every effective with lung complaints – take the SONA listed in part I of this book.
HERBALS	Thyme, Echinacea, Garlic.
LIFESTYLE CHANGES	If you suffer frequently from respiratory problems take up swimming, especially breaststroke. This is an excellent exercise for those with lung disorders.

RESPIRATORY SYSTEM RULE NO 2

Ginger destroys influenza viruses.
Prevention is better than cure so experiment and make ginger tea and
use liberally in home-made dishes

COMMON COLD

The common cold is an acute (short term) viral infection of the upper
respiratory tract which often causes runny nose, sore throat, and
malaise. Sore throat is sometimes a symptom of a more serious
condition distinct from the common cold that may require medical
diagnosis and treatment with appropriate antibiotics. If antibiotics are
required the treatment should be followed up by a course of probiotics
to replace the good gut flora.

Sugar, dietary fat, and alcohol have been reported to affect the immune
system negatively, though no specific information is yet available as to
how much these foods may actually affect the course of the common
cold.

Vitamin C and zinc have been tested rigorously over the past years in
common cold trials and have both been raked primary supplements
for the common cold and immune system generally. A review of
twenty-one placebo-controlled studies using 1–8mg of vitamin C
found that 'in each of the twenty-one studies, vitamin C reduced the
duration of episodes and the severity of the symptoms of the common
cold by an average of 23 per cent'.[253] The optimum amount of vitamin
C to take for cold treatment remains in debate but 1–3 grams per day
is commonly used and is generally supportive of much of the scientific
literature.

Zinc has many functions in connection with the common cold, it
interferes with viral replication in test tubes; may interfere with the
ability of the virus to enter the cells of the body; may help immune
cells to fight a cold; and may relieve cold symptoms by affecting
prostaglandin metabolism.[254] Certain zinc lozenges have been helpful
to adult cold sufferers though this effect has not been reported in
children. Most successful studies have used zinc gluconate or zinc
gluconate-glycine lozenges containing 15–25mg of zinc per lozenge.

An analysis of the major zinc trials has claimed that evidence for efficacy is 'still lacking'. However, despite a lack of *statistical* significance, this compilation of data from six double blind trials found that people assigned to zinc had a 50 per cent decreased risk of still having symptoms after one week compared with those given placebo. Zinc lozenges should not be taken long term but rather on the onset of a cold and stopped when symptoms have disappeared. The best effect is obtained when lozenges are used at the first sign of a cold when up to ten lozenges per day can be taken for the first few days.

In traditional herbal medicine, goldenseal root is often taken with echinacea. Two alkaloids in the root (berberine and canadine) have an anti-microbial and mild immune-stimulating effect. Goldenseal soothes irritated mucous membranes in the throat making it useful to those experiencing a sore throat with their cold.

Herbal supplements can play a role in the long-term attempts to strengthen the immune system and fight infections. Adaptogens, which include Siberian ginseng, Asian ginseng, astragalus and schisandra are though to help keep various body systems including the immune system functioning optimally. Another immune stimulant, boneset helps fight minor viral infections, such as the common cold.

Herbs high in mucilage such as slippery elm and marshmallow are often helpful for symptomatic relief of coughs and irritated throats. Mullein has expectorant properties which accounts for this herb's historical use as a remedy for the respiratory system particularly in cases of irritating coughs with bronchial congestion.

Eucalyptus oil is often used in a steam inhalation to help clear nasal and sinus congestion and is said to function in a fashion similar to that of menthol by acting on receptors in the mucosa, leading to a reduction in the symptoms of, for example, nasal stuffiness.

Treatment of colds is to encourage elimination through all channels so that eliminations through only one channel do not become excessive.

RECOMMENDATIONS FOR COMMON COLD

DIET	A light diet is recommended – high in liquids.
INCREASE	Hot water with lemon and Manuka honey. Hot water with apple cider vinegar, and Manuka honey Herbal teas. Fruit and homemade thin vegetable soups. Ginger tea.
DECREASE	Dairy foods, meat, all 'heavy' foods, alcohol, everything refined.
SUPERFOODS	Manuka honey, Chlorophyll, Bee Pollen, liquorice.
SUPPLEMENTS	Vitamin C taken throughout the day – every two hours for the first few days of a cold. Zinc, Garlic capsules,
HERBALS	Echinacea, Siberian ginseng, Asian ginseng, Goldenseal root
LIFESTYLE CHANGES	Treat yourself to a sauna and treat your cold at the same time. Take eucalyptus oil to add to the sauna water and also use as a steam inhalation.

SINUSITIS

Sinusitis is an upper respiratory condition that involves the inflammation of the accessory nasal sinuses. There are four pairs of sinuses in the human skull that helps circulate moist air through the nasal passages. The common cold is the most prevalent predisposing factor to sinusitis. Acute sinusitis typically causes symptoms of nasal congestion and a thick yellow or green discharge. Other symptoms include tenderness and pain over the sinuses, frontal headaches, and sometimes chills, fever and pressure in the area of the sinuses. Chronic sinusitis differs slightly in that symptoms can be milder and may only include postnasal drip, bad breath and an irritating dry cough. Hay fever, environmental triggers, unrelated hay fever, food allergens, and dental infections can also lead to sinusitis.

The typical patient with chronic sinusitis characteristically follows an acid-forming diet, having an excess of starches and dairy products and lacking in sufficient raw green vegetables. This type of diet causes an increase in the amount of mucus produced by the body and favours tissue congestion. According to some studies, 25 per cent of people with sinusitis have environmental allergies.[262] Although food allergies may contribute to the problem, many researchers believe food allergies only rarely *cause* sinusitis. If other treatment approaches are unsuccessful people with sinusitis may choose to work with a nutrition and allergy therapist to evaluate what, if any, effect elimination of certain foods and other allergens might have on reducing their symptoms.

Histamine is associated with increased nasal and sinus congestion. In one study vitamin C supplementation of 1g three times a day reduced histamine levels in people with either high histamine levels or low blood levels of vitamin C. [263] Another study found that 2g of vitamin C helped protect individuals exposed to a histamine challenge.

Bromelain, an enzyme derived from pineapple, has been reported to relieve symptoms of acute sinusitis. In a double blind study comparing the use of bromelain with placebo, those patients who took bromelain reported good to excellent results compared with the placebo group. Other double blind research has shown that bromelain reduces symptoms of sinusitis.[264]

In a preliminary trial supplementation of 250mg of pantothenic acid twice a day was demonstrated to help most clients suffering from allergic rhinitis, a significant predisposing factor for sinusitis. However, research has yet to investigate the effects of pantothenic acid supplementation with people who have sinusitis.

Herbs that have proved useful are stinging nettles and eucalyptus. An isolated double blind study compared the use of free dried stinging nettles with placebo. In that one-week trial, 300mg of stinging nettles taken twice per day led to moderate effectiveness among 58 per cent of those in the treatment group compared with only 37 per cent in the placebo group.

Eucalyptus oil is often used in a steam inhalation to help clear nasal and sinus congestion. Eucalyptus oil is said to function in a fashion similar to that of menthol by acting on receptors in the nasal mucosa, leading to a reduction in the symptoms of, for example, nasal stuffiness.[256]

A mucus cleansing diet is recommended for clients suffering with sinusitis. This includes a high quantity liquid diet for up to three days if that can be tolerated. A mucus cleansing diet would comprise of lemon or grapefruit juice every morning either alone or with warm water. A mid-morning snack would comprise of juiced vegetables such as carrot or carrot and celery. Lunch would comprise as many onions to be eaten either boiled or steamed with a citrus fruit for dessert. More vegetable juice in the afternoon. More onions for an evening meal and garlic capsules. This is very effective but difficult to follow but most clients suffering chronic sinusitis are willing to try anything for relief. A nutritional therapist will give you a more complete mucus cleansing diet if you want to follow this course of action. Most diets of this type start with two or three days of cleansing followed by additional foods being introduced in a particular sequence.

RESPIRATORY SYSTEM RULE NO 3

Japanese tests have found that a substance called lentinan in Shiitake mushrooms fights influenza viruses better than a prescription antiviral drug.

RECOMMENDATIONS FOR SINUSITIS

DIET	Mucus cleaning diet. Mostly liquids for 2 days followed by a raw fruit and vegetables for a further 2 days then a light, low protein diet, avoiding dairy products.
INCREASE	Citrus fruits, vegetable juices, boiled and steamed onions, water.
DECREASE	Red meat, all dairy products.
SUPERFOODS	Alfalfa, Algae, Barley Grass, Bee Pollen, Liquorice and Medicinal Mushrooms.
SUPPLEMENTS	SONA of Vitamin A Vitamin B complex with no less than 25mg of the B vitamins. Vitamin C minimum 1 g daily.
HERBALS	Garlic, Fenugreek and Black cohosh.
LIFESTYLE CHANGES	Daily exercise walking especially – don't make it too easy. Inhalations using eucalyptus or oil of pine.

GENERAL RECOMMENDATIONS FOR
THE RESPIRATORY SYSTEM

DIET **FOODS TO SUPPORT**	Hot water with lemon and Manuka honey. Hot water with apple cider vinegar, and Manuka honey Herbal teas. Fruit and homemade thin vegetable soups. Ginger tea. Oily Fish, hot chilli peppers, horseradish. Always a light diet – as fluid as possible.
FOODS TO AVOID	Milk and dairy products
SUPERFOODS	Manuka honey Liquorice Chlorophyll Bee Pollen
SUPPLEMENTS	Vitamin C Zinc N-acetyl cysteine (NAC), Thymus glandular, Co-Q-10, Fish Oils Vitamin A
HERBAL REMEDIES	Marshmallow, Garlic capsules.
LIFESTYLE CHANGES	Regular swimming – especially breaststroke. Saunas – using eucalyptus or pine oil in the sauna water or use these oils as steam inhalations. If you are feeling really brave, try hydrotherapy by alternating hot and cold showers to stimulate respiration and circulation. Treat yourself to a visit to a health spa where they will have a wide range of therapeutic hydrotherapy treatments to stimulate the respiratory and circulatory systems.

THE SKELETAL SYSTEM

What is the Skeletal system?

The skeletal system is the system of the body offering support and protection by several types of connective tissue — cartilage, bone and dense connective tissue.

Main functions

The skeletal system performs several basic functions.

Support	The skeleton provides a framework for the body, and as such, it supports soft tissues and provides a point of attachment for many muscles.
Protection	Many internal organs are protected from injury by the skeleton. For example, the brain is protected by the cranial bones, the spinal cord by the vertebrae, the heart and lungs by the rib cage and internal reproductive organs by the pelvic bones.
Movement facilitation	Bones serve as levers to which muscles are attached. When the muscles contract, bones acting as levers and movable joints acting as fulcrums produce movement.
Mineral Storage	Bones store several minerals that can be distributed to other parts of the body upon demand. The principal stored minerals are calcium and phosphorus.
Storage of blood cell-producing cells	Red marrow in certain bones is capable of producing blood cells. Red marrow produces red blood cells, some white blood cells, and platelets.

What does the Skeletal system actually do?

As the framework for the whole body the skeletal system provides attachments for muscles, and an important store for vital minerals. It is a system usually forgotten about within nutritional therapy, but such an important one to bear in mind.

Dietary influences affecting the skeletal system

Physical fitness is the major determinant of the fitness of the skeletal system. Calcium, magnesium, boron, and vitamin K all have important roles to play in the health of the bones. The aches and pains, stooped posture, loss of teeth and bone fractures of osteoporosis and an elevation in blood pressure were once called the inevitable result of 'old age'. It is now recognised that these diseases are influenced by a lifetime of habits. The choices a person makes about diet, exercise and other health habits will have an effect on whether the bones remain strong and upright or become porous and hunched, and whether the blood pressure and heart will remain healthy.

COMMON DISORDERS

GOUT

Gout is a common arthritic condition usually associated with a high acidic diet as in an excess of meat, dairy, and alcohol.

The small joints of the fingers but especially the toes are usually affected. For a change gout is ten times more common in men than women, who tend to have the disease after the menopause. The most characteristic feature of gout is that it is usually accompanied by an increase in the amount of uric acid in the blood. Uric acid is the end product of the body's metabolism of substances, called purines. These are compounds that form part of the RNA and DNA of the nuclei of the body's cells. Not all purines however are converted into uric acid in the body; the caffeine in tea and coffee, and theobromine in cocoa and chocolate, are purines that do not produce uric acid. Since the pruines that do produce uric acid are found chiefly in cells, especially animal cells, the purine rich foods are liver, kidney, shellfish and fish roes because these foods have an unusually high proportion of cells.

Recommendations are to reduce alcohol, avoid all purine rich foods, drink plenty of water to flush out and promote excretion of the uric acid and significantly reduce refined foods. Good supplements are celery seed which is thought to help eliminate uric acid through the kidneys and cherries or other sources of anthocyanidians which are thought to help decrease inflammation and uric acid levels. Oxalic acid, found in rhubarb, sorrel and spinach is another food residue that can often exacerbate the problem so these foods too should be avoided.

RECOMMENDATIONS FOR GOUT

DIET	A general well balanced diet taking foods from all the main food groups, carbohydrates, low fat proteins, and essential fatty acids. Do not over eat.
INCREASE	Green leafy vegetables and drink at least 1 pint of water every day – up to 1 litre would be better.
DECREASE	Avoid rich foods including liver, kidney, red meat, game and fish roes. Too much fruit consumption or the use of fruit sugar (fructose) might also aggravate gout.
SUPERFOODS	Alfalfa, Spirulina, Chorella and blue-green algae – rotate each month. Bee Pollen.
SUPPLEMENTS	Vitamin C – up to 3g daily – to increase loss of uric acid via the kidneys. Zinc up to 15mg daily. Bone mineral complex (rich in alkaline-forming calcium and magnesium).
HERBALS	None specifically
LIFESTYLE CHANGES	Lose weight if you are overweight. Avoid alcohol completely. Avoid lead, cadmium, mercury and aluminium.

SKELETAL SYSTEM RULE NO 1

Daily weight bearing exercise will strengthen bones throughout your life

OSTEOPOROSIS – BRITTLE BONE DISEASE

This condition is often referred to as the 'silent epidemic' as until you actually fracture a bone, you don't know you've got it. The literal meaning of osteoporosis is 'porous bone'. It is a condition in which the bones may become brittle and liable to fracture.[100] The bone tissue of an adult is usually at its most dense between the ages of 30 and 35 years.[101] After this age the bone density will decline naturally.[102] Bone loss tends to be greater in women than in men, primarily due to increased bone loss during the menopausal and post-menopausal years. This is due to hormonal changes, especially the loss of the protective effects of oestrogen, as levels decline. The whole skeleton may be affected by osteoporosis, however, bone loss is usually greatest in the spine, hips, and ribs.

Increasing bone mass during adolescence through sufficient calcium intake could decrease the risk of osteoporosis in later life. It may also be beneficial to take magnesium and vitamin D supplements because these two nutrients are involved in the uptake and utilisation of calcium. Studies have examined vitamin D and calcium supplementation and found that it may moderately reduce bone loss.[103]

There is evidence to support that DHEA levels may be a factor in age-related bone loss. DHEA is manufactured by the adrenal glands, but it is also one of the four major hormones produced by the ovaries; the others are oestrogen, progesterone and testosterone. DHEA has many functions, one being a precursor hormone, which almost certainly results in a beneficial influence on osteoporosis. DHEA can be converted by the body into other hormones including oestrogen and testosterone, both of which play a role in prevention of bone loss. In a study of post-menopausal women, administering DHEA increased serum levels of both testosterone and oestrogens.

An osteoporosis-prevention diet should restrict refined sugar, caffeine, and alcohol and protein and salt intake should be moderate. There is evidence that some individuals lose calcium from their body if they ingest too much salt. Whole grains should be used instead of refined grains because refining of grains results in substantial losses of many of the vitamins and minerals needed to maintain healthy bones. All fizzy drinks which contain excessive amounts of phosphorus should also be avoided, since too much phosphorus may adversely affect calcium metabolism.

Do not forget that bone is a living tissue that needs a wide range of nutritional needs. Failure to meet any one of a number of different nutritional requirements could promote osteoporosis.

SKELETAL SYSTEM RULE NO 2

An alkaline forming diet rich in magnesium will keep calcium in the bone where we want it. An acidic diet will encourage calcium to leave the bones

---

RECOMMENDATIONS FOR OSTEOPOROSIS

DIET	Natural diet, low in saturated fats and refined foods.
INCREASE:	Magnesium rich foods, such as green leafy vegetables, plenty of fruit. Protein choices should be of the low saturated fat variety, chicken, turkey, fish, tofu.
DECREASE	A protein rich diet may be an underlying cause of osteoporosis, as excess may leach calcium from bones.
SUPERFOODS	
SUPPLEMENTS	**Lysine** — thought to enhance intestinal calcium absorption [104] **Vitamin C** — associated with higher bone mineral density in early post menopausal women [105] **Boron** — which has been shown to reduce losses of dietary calcium.
HERBALS	Black Cohosh
LIFESTYLE CHANGES	Weight bearing exercise – no matter what age you are

OSTOARTHRITIS

Osteoarthritis is a common disease that develops when linings of joints fail to maintain normal structure, leading to pain and decreased mobility. It is associated with aging and injury — it used to be called 'wear and tear' arthritis.

Solanine is a substance found in nightshade plants, including tomatoes, white potato, peppers (except black pepper) and eggplant. In theory, if not destroyed in the intestines solanine could be toxic. A horticulturist, Dr. Normal Childers, hypothesized that some people with osteoarthritis may not be able to destroy solanine in the gut, leading to some absorption resulting in osteoarthritis. Eliminating solanine from the diet has been reported to bring relief to some arthritis sufferers in preliminary research.[294][295] An uncontrolled survey of people avoiding nightshade plants revealed that 28 per cent claimed to have a 'marked positive response' and another 44 per cent a 'positive response' Researchers have never put this to a strict clinical test. However, the treatment continues to be used by many nutritional therapists with people who have osteoarthritis.

Glucosamine sulphate (GS) a nutrient derived from seashells, contains a building block needed for the repair of joint cartilage and has significantly reduced symptoms of osteoarthritis in uncontrolled and single blind trials. Many double blind studies have also reported efficacy. All published clinical investigations on the effects of glucosamine sulfate in people with osteoarthritis report statistically significant improvement. Most research trials use 500mg GS taken three times per day. Benefits from glucosamine sulphate generally become evident after three to eight weeks of treatment. Continued supplementation is needed in order to maintain benefits.

Chondroitin sulphate (CS) is a major component of the lining of joints. In structure, chrondroitin sulphate is related to several molecules of glucosamine sulphate attached to each other. Levels of chondroitin sulphate have been reported to be reduced in joint cartilage affected by osteoarthritis. It has been found that both substances are required to ease the symptoms of osteoarthritis and supplements are now available that contain both glucosamine sulphate and chondroitin which are having beneficial results.

S-adenosyl methionine (SAMe) possesses anti-inflammatory pain relieving and tissue healing properties that may help protect the health of the joints.[296] [297] Double blind reports studying effects in people with osteoarthritis have consistently shown that SAMe increase the formation of healthy tissue and reduces pain, stiffness, and swelling better than a placebo and equal to drugs such as ibuprofen. On the basis of outcomes reported in published research, 400mg taken three times per day appears to be the optimal intake of SAMe.

People who have osteoarthritis and eat high levels of antioxidants from food have been reported to exhibit a much slower rate of joint deterioration, particularly in the knees, compared with people eating foods containing lower levels of antioxidants. Of the individual antioxidants, only vitamin E has been studied in controlled trials. Vitamin E has reduced symptoms of osteoarthritis in both single and double blind research. In several trials, 400–600ius of vitamin E per day has been used.

Herbs that may be useful are Boswellia which has a unique anti-inflammatory action, much like conventional non-steroidal anti-inflammatory drugs (NSAIDs) used by many for inflammatory conditions.[298] Clinical studies in humans are lacking but is used by many nutritional therapists. Unlike NSAIDs, however, long-term use of boswellia does not led to irritation or ulceration of the stomach.

RECOMMENDATIONS FOR OSTEOARTHRITIS

DIET	A whole food approach to food where quality is more important than quantity. Plenty of fruits, vegetables, nuts and seeds with adequate essential fatty acids, low-fat protein, and plenty of water.
INCREASE	Green leafy vegetables and oily fish.
DECREASE	Members of the nightshade family – tomatoes, white potato, peppers (except black pepper) and eggplant. Everything refined – especially white bread and flour, confectionery, and alcohol. Also red meat, eggs if you are eating in excess of 6 a week and all chemicals.
SUPERFOODS	Super Sprouts, Medicinal mushrooms, Bee Pollen and Barley Grass.
SUPPLEMENTS	MSM – a naturally occurring source of sulphur. Chondroitin sulphate and glucosamine sulphate in one supplements. SAMe, Vitamin E.
HERBALS	Boswellia and Black Cohosh
LIFESTYLE CHANGES	Check you do not have any food or chemical allergies as these are sometimes connected to all types of arthritis. Obesity is a risk factor for osteoarthritis of weight bearing joints. Weight loss is thought by arthritis experts to be of potential benefit, especially at reducing pain levels.

OSTEOMALACIA

Osteomalacia is a deficiency of Vitamin D, combined with a deficiency of calcium. It is the adult form of rickets. Especially prone to the disease are women who have repeated pregnancies and breast fed their babies. With these women their own bones become depleted of calcium causing weakness. Lack of exposure to sunlight is a contributory factor.

The few foods than contain vitamin D include egg yolks, butter, vitamin D-fortified milk, and fish liver oils,. Calcium is found in dairy products, sardines, salmon (canned with edible bones) leafy vegetables, and tofu. Pure vegetarians may use supplements instead of eggs and dairy as sources for both calcium and vitamin D.

Direct exposure of the skin to sunlight stimulates the body to manufacture vitamin D. However, both clothes and the use of sunscreen prevent the ultraviolet light that triggers the formation of vitamin D from reaching the skin. Depending upon the latitude, sunlight during the winter may not produce enough ultraviolet light to promote adequate vitamin D production. At other times during the year even thirty minutes of exposure per day will usually lead to large increases in the amount of vitamin D made.

SKELETAL SYSTEM RULE NO 3

Is your calcium being absorbed?
Alcohol, caffeine, some medications, high dietary protein and inactivity all decrease calcium absorption – so take care yours is getting through.

RECOMMENDATIONS FOR OSTEOMALACIA

DIET	A general diet covering all the main food groups, carbohydrates, low fat proteins and essential fatty acids. This would include nuts and seeds.
INCREASE	Oily fish – sardines salmon, herring, tuna and mackerel at least three times each week. The bones of the sardines and salmon (if tinned) should also be eaten. Vitamin D by increasing green leafy vegetables, tofu and small amounts of eggs, butter.
DECREASE	All refined, denatured foods, all chemicals, alcohol, white bread, flour and additives.
SUPERFOODS	Spirulina, Medicinal mushrooms, Barley Grass
SUPPLEMENTS	Multivitamin and mineral Vitamin D
HERBALS	None specifically
LIFESTYLE CHANGES	Expose arms, face and legs to sunshine for at least 30 minutes every day in summer and take a supplement in the winter.

GENERAL RECOMMENDATIONS FOR THE SKELETAL SYSTEM

DIET	
FOODS TO SUPPORT	Green leafy vegetables, all alkaline forming foods. Low fat dairy foods
FOODS TO AVOID	Purine rich foods, seafood, liver, fish roe, alcohol, all refined foods. Avoid alcohol, caffeine, a high protein diet, as all these can disrupt calcium absorption.
SUPERFOODS	Spirulina, Chlorella and Blue-Green Algae Watercress, Bee Pollen and Barley Grass
SUPPLEMENTS	MSM – a naturally occurring source of organic sulphur. SAMe Vitamin E. Magnesium and Calcium in a good ratio Glucosamine Sulfate with Chondroitin Lysine Vitamin C Boron
HERBAL REMEDIES	Herbal formula for the skeletal system: This formula is designed to provide nutrition for the bones, muscles and cartilage. Papaya, Parsley, Pineapple, Valerian, liquorice and Ma Huang.
LIFESTYLE CHANGES	Weight bearing exercises every day – these include walking, jogging, running.

URINARY AND DETOXIFICATION SYSTEMS

What are the Urinary and Detoxification systems?

Two kidneys, two ureters, one urinary bladder and a single urethra make up the urinary system. Other organs of detoxification are the liver, lungs and skin which also play an important part in removing toxins from our bodies.

Main function:

The primary function of the urinary system is to help keep the body in homeostasis by controlling the composition of volume of blood. The functions of the other organs are to eliminate unwanted toxins from the body.

What do the Urinary and Detoxification systems actually do?

The two kidneys of the urinary system removes and restores selected amounts of water and solutes. The kidneys regulate the composition and volume of the blood and remove wastes from the blood in the form of urine. The general functions of the kidneys are the removal of urea from bloodstream and the regulation of the body's fluids by controlling the water and mineral ion concentration of the blood.

The liver is the largest gland in the body and has many important functions in the metabolism of proteins, fats and carbohydrates. In its capacity as an organ of detoxification, it is responsible for detoxifying harmful toxic waste, synthetic hormones and drugs and excreting them in bile or through the kidneys.

Dietary influences affecting the urinary and detoxification systems

As you may expect, water is the key issue with this system. Water is needed on a regular basis to keep the kidneys in good working order. Other fluids can cause problems. Fizzy drinks, coffee and tea all have a detrimental effect on the system. Excessive use of alcohol however, has the strongest influence over the urinary and detoxification systems. Alcohol is a serious health threat that only provides intoxication and dehydration, and may upset blood sugar levels, as it is a chemical cousin of sugar. It can be classed as an anti-nutrient, which means that it uses up more nutrients than it provides. It can severely damage the liver, and puts excess toxic load on the body giving the kidneys extra work to do along the way.

DETOX/URINARY SYSTEM RULE NO 1
Drink at least 1 liter of water every day

COMMON DISORDERS
INCONTINENCE

Incontinence is the lack of voluntary control over micturition – passing urine. This is usually in very small amounts accompanying coughing, sneezing, laughing, walking, running, lifting or any sudden shock or strain. In infants about two years old and under, incontinence is normal because neurons to the external sphincter muscle are not completely developed. Infants' void whenever the urinary bladder is sufficiently distended to arouse a reflex stimulus. Proper training overcomes incontinence if the latter is not cause by emotional stress or irritation of the urinary bladder.

Involuntary micturition in the adult may occur as a result of repeated births, failure to do prenatal and postnatal exercises, poor pelvic floor tone, injury to the spinal nerves controlling the urinary bladder, irritation due to abnormal constituents in urine, or disease of the urinary bladder. It is a condition that can be very stressful and embarrassing.

It is most common in women that have had children, but in women who have never had a child, it is much less common. Weak abdominal tone, obesity, and lack of pelvic muscle tone are the major causative factors involved in these cases.

Surgery is sometimes undertaken to correct incontinence. However, surgery can be avoided if proper exercises are regularly taken, especially before pregnancy. Pelvic exercises must begin during early pregnancy or before, and continued just after the birth for at least three months or longer. Dr. Arnold Kegal, a professor of obstetrics and gynecology at the University of California in Los Angeles developed a series of pelvic floor exercises that are still used very much today. They are commonly known as the 'Kegal' exercises. Here are two for you to try.

1. Practice slowing urine flow and eventually stopping it to gain a sense of which muscles are involved. Later, practice stopping urine flow, hold for 1 to 2 seconds and repeat six to eight times as you urinate. Eventually you should be able to stop urine flow quickly, without any leakage and slowly relax the pelvic floor muscles in stages from full contraction to full relaxation.
2. Use the same muscles that you mastered the control of in the first exercise to contract the pelvic floor throughout the day. Do this whenever and wherever possible. This may be repeated six to eight times during each session and 50 to 100 times a day. Hold the contraction 2 to 5 seconds and then relax.

When doing these exercises, do not hold your breath, bear down (thus pushing down on the pelvic floor) or contract the buttocks, inner thighs, or abdominal muscles. It is best to learn to localise the contraction to the pelvic floor muscles entirely. Do no exhaust the pelvic floor muscles in the early stages. Do only as many contractions at a time as you can do at your maximum contraction and then two to three more. As contractions weaken discontinue at that time and build the muscle strength slowly, as is done with any other muscular exercise.

URINARY/DETOX SYSTEMS RULE NO 2
Never ignore the calls of nature.
When you need to go to the toilet — go — it may save you future problems.

RECOMMENDATIONS FOR INCONTINENCE

DIET	A whole food approach to food where quality is more important than quantity. Plenty of fruits and vegetables, low-fat protein, and plenty of water.
INCREASE	Nothing specifically – general good food like fruit and vegetables.
DECREASE	Nothing specifically – general recommendations. All junk food, red meat, alcohol.
SUPERFOODS	Alfalfa, and Barley Grass
SUPPLEMENTS	None specifically
HERBALS	None specifically
LIFESTYLE CHANGES	Take up the Kegal exercises – whatever your age and however serious the problem, it is never too late to start. Alternatively swimming – breast stroke/frog kick Bicycling Alternate hot and cold sitz baths – *not if pregnant*

URINARY TRACT INFECTIONS

Urinary tract infections (UTIs) are infections of the kidney, bladder and urethra, which are under the control of the immune system. They are generally triggered by bacteria and are more common with any partial blockage of the urinary tract. Many people have recurring bouts of urinary tract infections.

Cystitis, is probably the most common of the UTIs and describes inflammation of the bladder and/or urethra. Infection or bruising or irritation or a combination of these may cause it. The urethra is where you will feel much of the pain of cystitis. If the attack does turn out to be caused by an infection, and is not treated, it can spread up to the kidneys (via the bladder and the ureters) and produce a more serious infection. The most common symptoms are a burning pain whenever you pass water, a frequent and urgent need to pass water, even though when you try there is hardly any (or no) urine, and needing to get up often at night to pass water.

There are many dietary changes, supplement and herbal recommendations for these conditions, and some very interesting studies have been done in this field. One such study had healthy volunteers ingest a large amount (100 grams) of refined sugar, after which the ability of their white blood cells to destroy bacteria was impaired for at least five hours.[197.] Ingestion of excessive amounts of alcohol has also shown to suppress the immune system[198] whereas reducing the intake of dietary fat stimulates immunity.[199] For these reasons recommendations can be given to reduce sugar, alcohol and fat during an acute infection and for prevention of future recurrences.

Optimal levels of vitamin C are often recommended by nutritional therapists for acute UTIs as well as long-standing supplementation for individuals who are prone to recurrent infections. Although no control studies have demonstrated the effectiveness of vitamin C for this purpose, this vitamin has been shown to inhibit the growth of *E.coli*, the most common bacterial cause of urinary tract infections and in addition, ingestion of 4g or more of vitamin C per day results in a slight acidisation of the urine[200] creating an 'unfriendly' environment for certain bacteria.

Since the immune system requires many nutrients in order to function properly, many people take a multivitamin/mineral supplement for 'insurance'. In one double blind study, healthy elderly people using such a supplement for one year showed improvements in certain measures of immune function, as well as a significant reduction in the total number of infections (including non urinary tract infections).[201]

There are numerous herbal remedies for urinary tract infections the most popular and well known being cranberry and modern research has confirmed the benefits of cranberry for the prevention of UTIs. Drinking 10–16 ounces of unsweetened or lightly sweetened cranberry juice is recommended for prevention and as part of the treatment of urinary tract infections. In a double blind study, elderly women who drank 10 ounces of cranberry juice per day had a decrease in the amount of bacteria in their urine.[201] In another study elderly residents of a nursing home consumed either four ounces of cranberry juice or six capsules containing concentrated cranberry daily for thirteen months. During that time, the number of UTIs decreased by 25 per cent.[202] Researchers have suggested two possible ways in which cranberry is effective against UTIs. First, cranberry prevents *E.coli*, the bacteria that causes most urinary tract infections, from attaching to the walls of the bladder.[203] Second, cranberry contains hippuric acid, a compound that has been found to have antibiotic activity.[204] However, cranberry should not be used as a substitute for antibiotics in the treatment of acute UTIs.

Goldenseal is reputed to help treat many types of infections. It contains berberine, an alkaloid that may prevent UTIs in the same way as cranberry, by inhibiting bacteria from adhering to the wall of the bladder. Goldenseal and other plants containing berberine such as Oregon grape can therefore help in the treatment and prevention of urinary tract infections.

Herbs that work by increasing urinary volume, thereby helping to flush bacteria out of the urinary tract, could be added as a tincture to water. Herbs with this function include Asparagus *(Asparagus officinalis)*, Birch *(Betula supp.)* Goldenrod *(Solidago virgaurea)*, Juniper and Nettle.

DETOX/URINARY SYSTEM RULE NO 3

Alcohol is classed as an anti-nutrient,
which means that it uses up more nutrients than it provides.
<u>Maximum</u> is 14 units per week for women
and 21 units per week for men
spread out over the week – and not saved up for the weekends!!

RECOMMENDATIONS FOR URINARY TRACT INFECTIONS

DIET	A diet high fruits and vegetables to boost immune system.
INCREASE	Kiwi fruit, strawberries, oranges, red, green and yellow peppers, and asparagus.
DECREASE	Sugar, saturated fats, and alcohol.
SUPERFOODS	Alfalfa, Algae, Barley Grass, Bee Pollen, Honey, and Medicinal Mushrooms.
SUPPLEMENTS	A good multivitamin and mineral with additional vitamin C to bowel tolerance for one month then decrease. Propolis — a natural anti-biotic which helps to kill harmful bacteria.
HERBALS	Cranberry (as tablets or juice), Goldenseal.
LIFESTYLE CHANGES	Water intake of $1\frac{1}{2}$ liters every day should become a habit.

WATER RETENTION/ODEMA AND FLUID BALANCE IN THE BODY

Abnormal accumulation of fluid beneath the skin is known as odema. There are two basic types of water retention. The first is when water is retained in the cells, thus causing swelling and a spongy feeling. The other is when the blood capillaries are not working efficiently. Congestive heart failure and pre-eclampsia of pregnancy are also connected with fluid retention but these causes must be medically treated.

Many people, especially women suffer from fluid retention. The usual symptoms are swelling of hands, ankles, feet, face abdomen, or other areas of the body, premenstrual syndrome, headaches, and leg ulcers.

Fluid Balance in the Body explained: Water makes up about 70 per cent of the adult human body i.e. about 46 liters in a 70kg man. Some lie outside the cells called extracellular fluid (16 liters) and a large part is within the cell called intracellular fluid (30 liters).

The body maintains a state of homeostasis at all times. Homeostasis is the maintenance of a constant internal environment in the body. It is completing thousands of chemical reactions every second to keep us alive, and a vital part of the homeostasis mechanism is the regulation of body fluids.

In health the total amount of body water (and salt) is kept reasonably constant in spite of wide fluctuations in daily intake. A balance is struck between fluid intake and fluid output. Fluid intake is more than just the liquid we drink. We consume approximately 1000ml of liquid daily. In addition, 1200ml of 'liquid' also comes from the food we eat, 1500 from saliva, 2200ml is produced from plasma to assist the digestive system absorb nutrients, 1500ml comes from gastric juice, 800ml comes from bile, 1400ml comes from pancreatic juice, another 1500ml comes from intestinal juice and our body cells produce metabolic water of 400ml per day. So you see we have plenty of intake – but what about output?

We lose 150ml in feces, 450ml in sweat, 1500ml in urine, 500ml from the lungs, 150,000ml from kidney filtration (although 148,000ml of this is reabsorbed). So you can see intake and output are pretty well balanced.

Except in growth, convalescence or pregnancy – when new tissue is being formed – an increase or decrease in intake leads to an appropriate increase or decrease in output to maintain the balance. So what goes wrong? Why do so many people, especially women, suffer from fluid retention? It is connected with the endocrine system in that ADH – anti diuretic hormone secreted from the adrenal glands, gives chemical messages to the kidneys to either hold on to or release urine.

Any waste product the body makes during metabolism must be removed from the body. For example, carbon dioxide is a waste product from cell respiration and is expired in the air from our lungs.

In the same way water is a waste product from cell respiration and from the diet and is excreted in urine. Excretion of body wastes are carried out by the kidneys but the kidneys have several other functions, all concerned with maintaining the constant composition of the body fluids.

Fluid balance in the body is a complex issue. The best advice you can give anybody is to drink more water. It is so simple to do, but few actually meet the health guidelines of 1 liter daily. Many people think that by drinking more water they will make their situation worse, when the opposite is true.

As well as water itself, there are many foods that are natural diuretics and it is possible to lose many pounds of fluid over just a few days by incorporating these natural foods into your diet on a daily basis. These foods include: apples avocados, bananas, beans, beetroot, broccoli, cabbage, carrots, celery, oily fish (salmon, herring, mackerel, pilchards), lentils, liver, nuts & seeds, tomatoes, watercress and yoghurt.

Juicing is excellent for water retention and many interesting drinks can be made which will give very effective results. Try celery, parsley and radish juice, or beetroot juice with a little lemon, or apple on its own or mixed with a little lemon. Carrot and apple juice is a favourite and very beneficial for anyone with fluid retention. There are lots of books on the market with juicing recipes or if you really can't be bothered, find your nearest juice bar instead of the nearest wine bar – you will be pleased you did!

Coumarin is a bioflavonoid-like compound found in a variety of herbs, that has been used for odema. Both animal[127] and human[128] studies have found that coumarin can be beneficial in treating odema. Even odema after surgery (when lymphatic drainage is damaged) has been helped by coumarin. Alfalfa sprouts are a rich source of coumarin and comes high on the list of recommendations for reducing water retention.

Bilberries and blueberries are both rich in flavonoids and as such are excellent fruits for fluid retention. You can buy them frozen from most supermarkets. After defrosting, you can eat them as they are or warm them in the oven.

Herbal teas are also very beneficial for clients with water retention, as they are often rich in flavonoids and coumarin. Herbal teas are just that – herbal. Fennel, Comfrey, Clover Blossom, Nettle, Parsley, Chamomile, Peppermint, or any mixture of these. *Fruit* teas, are probably more beneficial than stimulant drinks such as coffee or tea, but they can also be very acidic and not as beneficial as the true herbal teas.

RECOMMENDATIONS FOR FLUID RETENTION

DIET	A low salt diet, otherwise balanced meals containing all the main food groups with low to medium protein intake.
INCREASE	Fruits and vegetables
DECREASE	Salt, salted nuts, smoked products,
SUPERFOODS	Rotate — Spirulina, Chlorella and Blue-Green Algae. in addition to Alfalfa
SUPPLEMENTS	Bioflavonoids – a mixed complex of 1,000mg daily
HERBALS	Goldenrod is considered to be one of the strongest herbal diuretics.[126] Quercetin and Ginkgo Biloba
LIFESTYLE CHANGES	Regular daily exercise — especially if occupation requires long period of sitting.

GENERAL RECOMMENDATIONS FOR THE URINARY SYSTEM

DIET **FOODS TO SUPPORT**	Eating adequate supplies of meat, milk, cheese, breads and cereals provide a good supply of amino acids and helps control bacterial growth.
FOODS TO AVOID	Citrus fruits and juices should be avoided
SUPERFOODS	Alfalfa, Rotate — Spirulina, Chlorella and Blue-Green Algae. Alfalfa, Barley Grass, Bee Pollen, Honey, and Medicinal Mushrooms.
SUPPLEMENTS	Vitamin C Kidney glandular tissue – gives support to the kidneys and helps rebuild damaged tissue Vitamin E, Proteolytic enzymes, Flaxseed and probiotics.
HERBAL REMEDIES	Ginkgo Biloba Golden rod – as a natural diuretic.
LIFESTYLE CHANGES	Drink plenty of water *every day*.and/or cranberry juice. Take up Kegal exercises if required in addition to daily regular exercise. Avoid alcohol or keep strictly to the maximum levels. Make AFDs part of your lifestyle – Alcohol Free Days and then work up to AFWs – Alcohol free weeks. It will be worth it.

PART III
PUTTING IT ALL TOGETHER

ESTABLISHING CURRENT DIET

The Consultation/Nutritional Questionnaire

The purpose of the nutrition consultation is to 'establish current diet' which is the main element for many accredited courses in nutrition.

In order to do this you need to ask specific questions. More importantly you need to know why you are asking the questions and how to interpret the answers.

The first thing you need to establish is what the client is actually consuming on a daily basis. You will therefore need a specific space on your consultation sheet for the clients to write down what they eat over a period of time. I ask for three days and one of these days to be a weekend day or non-working day. Leave a large area for this section, and additional space to write in snacks and drinks too. You need as much information as possible to enable you to establish an accurate overview of the client's current diet.

You will also need a separate question sheet for any supplementary information you may need from the client.

There are many other things to take into consideration when giving clients dietary advice. Knowing what the client is eating on a daily, or weekly basis, will only give you part of the picture. You must also take into consideration age, sex, any symptoms they have and the client's particular lifestyle.

Timing

It is important to establish the time of eating. Natural and healthy eating is regulated by feelings of hunger and satiety, but many people no longer tune in to these internal signals, or they confuse them with other feelings. For example, they may interpret anxiety as hunger. Or they may confuse feeling full with being fat.

Normalising the eating pattern should be considered as one of the most important aspects of helping your clients towards a healthy eating pattern and should be done in small steps.

The first step is to decide what time each day the client will eat three meals and two snacks. I normally give this as a task for the client to seriously think about. Give them plenty of time to really think about this, as once they have committed themselves to their times, I want them to stick to them – no matter what. They decide when they are going to eat.

These times can work around their family and work life so the timings may be different on a weekday to a weekend. Once established eating times have been set, the client should eat only during those times. They need to allow themselves only enough time to eat the meal or snack. A meal ordinarily should take no longer than thirty minutes to consume and a snack no more than fifteen minutes.

Initially, the client needn't worry about what they eat at each time period. Instead the focus is on eating within a regular schedule. In the client can establish this new eating pattern for 28 days – it will become a habit. The focus can then be on making healthier choices with regard to food. Eat at the planned times, even if you don't feel hungry. Don't skip meals or planned snacks, and try not to eat at other times. If you do slip and eat at an unplanned times just get back to the proper timings as soon as possible.

Try this exercise yourself. When you feel the benefits yourself of eating at a regular time, you will be in a much better position to advise your clients.

3 DAY FOOD DIARY

	DAY 1	DAY 2	DAY 3
Time	Breakfast	Breakfast	Breakfast
Time	Lunch	Lunch	Lunch
Time	Dinner	Dinner	Dinner
Time	Snack	Snack	Snack
Time	Snack	Snack	Snack
Time	Drinks	Drinks	Drinks
Time	Other	Other	Other

THE WEAKEST LINK QUESTIONNAIRE

To identify your client's weakest body system.

INSTRUCTIONS – questionnaire to be completed by therapist.

Ask every question and record with either a 'yes or 'no' answer.

It is important to ask all questions.

All answers carry one point except the skeletal, respiratory and nervous systems which all score 2 points for each yes answer.

At the end, add up each system separately and complete the 'totals' box.

Each section has a possible score of 10.

CARDIVASCULAR SYSTEM (1 point for each yes)   YES   NO

Are you more than 14lbs (7kgs) overweight?

Do you smoke more than 5 cigarettes a day?

Is there a history of heart disease in your family?

Do you have more than 2 alcoholic drinks a day?

Do you usually add salt to you food?

Do you eat red meat more than 5 times a week?

Do you use more than one spoon of sugar a day?

Do you do less than two hours exercise a week?

Is your blood pressure above 140/90?

Is your pulse after 15 minutes rest above 75?

Total scores for cardiovascular system

DIGESTIVE SYSTEM (1 point for each yes)   YES   NO

Do you suffer with constipation or diarrhoea?

Do you experience anal irritation?

Do you suffer from flatulence or bloating?

Do you occasionally use indigestion tablets?

Do you find it difficult digesting fatty foods?

Do you ever get a burning sensation in your stomach?

Are you prone to stomach upsets?

Do you use any type of butter or margarine on a daily basis?

Do you eat quickly/rush your food/eat under stress?

Do you normally eat at irregular times?

Total scores for digestive system

ENDOCRINE/REPRODUCTIVE SYSTEMS   YES   NO
   (1 point for each yes)

Are you taking or have you ever taken The Pill and/or HRT?

Have you ever had a miscarriage?

Do you suffer with any PMS symptoms?

Do you have difficulty in losing weight?

Do you suffer from lumpy breasts?

Do you suffer from breast tenderness?

Do you often feel tired during the day?

Do you often do 2 or 3 tasks simultaneously?

Do you have difficulty in getting to sleep?

Total scores for endocrine/reproductive systems

LYMPHATIC SYSTEM AND IMMUNITY   YES NO

(1 point for each yes)

Is there a history of cancer in your family?

Do you find it hard to shift an infection?

Do you sit still for several hours each day? work/TV

Do you avoid physical exercise?

Do you have cellulite?

Do you work harder than most people?

Do you feel guilty when relaxing?

Do you have a persistent need for achievement?

Are you especially competitive?

Have you taken antibiotics over the past 2 years?

Total scores for lymphatic and immunity systems

RESPIRATORY (2 marks each yes)   YES NO

Do you suffer from frequent bronchitis, asthma, colds & flu?

Do you smoke more than 5 cigarettes per day?

Do you live/work in a smoky atmosphere?

Do you live or work in a 'chemical' atmosphere?

(paint, thinners, petrol, fertilisers, hair sprays, colours etc.)

Do you eat your fruit and vegetables without washing?

Total scores for respiratory system

SKELETAL SYSTEM (2 marks for each yes)   **YES NO**

Do you consume more than 1 pint of milk per day?

Do you avoid weight-bearing exercise?

Do you eat *less than* 5 portions green leafy vegetables
and fruit *on a daily basis?*

Do you eat sweet, sugary, foods on most days?

Do you suffer with any type of arthritis?

Total scores for the skeletal system

URINARY/DETOXIFICTION SYSTEMS   **YES NO**
  (1 point for each yes)

Do you suffer with fluid retention?

Have you ever suffered with thrush or cystitis?

Do you suffer from chronic fatigue?

Do you have more than 2 alcoholic drinks a day?

Do you suffer with eczema or psoriasis?

Do you suffer from acne or poor skin condition?

Do you feel you have a sensitivity to chemicals?

Do you have any unexplained itching?

Do you drink more than 2 glasses of alcohol ***every day?***

Do you suffer with dull headaches?

Totals for the urinary/detoxification systems

NERVOUS SYSTEM (2 points for each yes)   **YES NO**

Do you suffer from any type of headache?

Do you suffer with migraine headaches

Do you suffer with 'panic attacks'?

Do you often find yourself irritable/jumpy?

Do you feel that you lose your temper easily?

Totals for the nervous system

MUSCULAR SYSTEM – ENERGY YES NO

(1 mark for each yes)

Is your energy less now than it used to be?

Do you avoid exercise due to tiredness?

Do you sweat a lot or get excessively thirsty?

Do you get dizzy or irritable if you don't eat often?

Do you often feel drowsy during the day?

Do you sometimes lose concentration?

Do you suffer with cramps?

Do you suffer with muscular aches and pains?

Do you have much injury through playing sport?

Do you drink less than 8 glasses of water every day?

TOTAL SCORES

	Total Yes answers	Total points
Cardiovascular System (1 point for each yes)		
Digestive System (1 point for each yes)		
Endocrine/Reproductive System (1 point for each yes)		
Lymphatic System and Immunity(2 points for each yes)		
Respiratory System 2 points for each yes)		
Skeletal System (2 points for each yes)		
Urinary and detoxification System (1 point for each yes)		
Nervous System (2 points for each yes)		
Muscular System and Energy (1 point for each yes)		

System with highest score ....

(If there is a tie between two systems – discuss with the client which system he/she would most like to work on. Alternatively, if you feel the client is able, they can start to support both systems for a faster return to optimum health.)

Once you have established the weakest system, go to the appropriate section in part II of the book and look under General Recommendations at the end of the chapter for suggestions for your client.

Agree with the client the course of action they want to take. They need to confirm in words with you that they are prepared to undertake the recommendations seriously to enhance their health and support their weakest system.

The dietary recommendations should always be made together with the superfoods. They may then add a lifestyle change and a supplement. Or they may decide on the herbal remedy and a lifestyle change. Everyone is different and different people will be drawn to different recommendations.

THE MISSING LINK QUESTIONS EXPLAINED

Here are some of the questions from the questionnaire and explanation why the question was asked. There are also some explanations to the clients answer, and your possible next course of action. You are trying to ascertain the causes of a symptom and there will always be more questions to ask in order to get to a possible explanation – working with nutrition is like being a detective.

CARDIOVASCULAR SYSTEM
Are you more than 14lbs/7kg overweight?
The answer to this should be no. Many of your clients will say yes. Assist and encourage them all you can to reduce. This will, without doubt help their heart work more efficiently.

Do you smoke more than 5 cigarettes a day?
Probably the worst activity as far as health is concerned is smoking. Assist and encourage client all you can to reduce and stop.

Is there a history of heart disease in your family?
Heart disease can be hereditary, but even with a yes answer, there is much the client can do for themselves. Stop smoking, regular gentle exercise and lots of green leafy vegetables, and cutting back on saturated fats. Heat disease is not inevitable even if it is hereditary in a family.

Do you have more than 2 alcoholic drinks a day?

Alcohol can be classed as an anti-nutrient. The more anti-nutrients we take into the body, the more nutrient deficient we become. Anyone who drinks more than 2 alcoholic drinks a day, would need an extra 500mg of Vitamin C a day compared to someone who did not drink.

Do you usually add salt to you food?

We do not need to add salt to our food. Excess sodium is associated with high blood pressure and fluid retention.

Do you eat red meat more than 5 times a week?

Eating meat more than 5 times a week is putting extra strain on the body. Not only are you ingesting the important protein content of the meat, but also the saturated fat that goes with it, not to mention the chemicals that were added to the feed of the animal that will be passed on to you. Growth hormones and antibiotics being just two.

Do you use more than one spoon of sugar a day?

Sugar in an anti-nutrient. If eaten in excess can contribute towards blood sugar problems, making you feel drowsy during the day and losing concentration. Zinc supplementation may improve your sense of taste, so reducing your need for sugar. Artificial sweeteners are a definite anti-nutrient and carcinogenic and clients should be made aware of this and strongly encouraged not to use them. If something must be added then choose $\frac{1}{2}$ teaspoon of Manuka honey.

Do you do less than two hours exercise a week?

Walking just $\frac{1}{2}$ hour daily (over and above your usual daily activities) may reduce heart diseases by up to 50%. The heart is a muscle and needs exercise like any other muscle.

Is your blood pressure above 140/90?

An obvious indicator that all is not right. Start now by exercising gently on a daily basis, just a 10-minute walk will help, reduce salt intake and increase consumption of green leafy vegetables. Its never too late to start looking after yourself.

Is your pulse after 15 minutes rest above 75?

Another indicator that all is not right. Same recommendations as blood pressure above.

DIGETIVE SYSTEM

Do you suffer with constipation or diarrhoea?

A yes answer would indicate that all is not well. Either condition is unpleasant and in indicator that the digestive system is compromised. Maybe the client is anxious or is eating too quickly under stressful conditions? There are many causes to be checked out here. You will need to ascertain if there are any food allergies or intolerances, exactly what is being eaten and when, how long has the client been suffering and has a visit been made to the doctor. IBS may be involved here.

Do you experience anal irritation?

If the answer is yes to this question, this could be linked with allergies and further investigations will have to be made.

Do you suffer from flatulence or bloating?

Many possibilities here for a yes answer. Investigate if they eat their food too quickly, thereby not allowing the digestive juices to act effectively – if so just by taking more time eating would make so much difference to their digestive system. Bloating could be a sign of candida albicans infestation or food allergy or intolerance. Look at their eating plan and see what you can pick up there. Check if they are drinking anything with their food. Liquid dilutes the digestive juices thereby making digestive enzymes less effective. Check out how many times they are eating wheat over one day and over one week. More than 7 times in a week? If so, this is too many. Try to encourage clients to have wheat a maximum of once a day for a start reducing to 3 times a week. Excessive wheat could be one reason for bloating. Suggest alternatives, oats, rice, barley, quinoa.

Do you occasionally use indigestion tablets?

If yes here – ask how often. If daily, this could be a serious matter. Many indigestion tables contain aluminum — of which there has been many studies to indicate a connection to Alzheimer's Disease. Nobody should need to take indigestion tablets daily. You could recommend taking a digestive enzyme supplement instead. This will assist in breaking down the food and helping digestion, and so avoiding the need to take the indigestion tablet.

Do you find it difficult digesting fatty foods?

This is usually a liver/gallbladder problem. Many clients have their gallbladders removed and are given no dietary advice. They have remained on their existing diet because they haven't been told otherwise, and hence find it extremely difficult to digest fatty food. Lecithin supplementation may be the answer. Sprinkled on to food it breaks down the fat content of food making it much more digestible Stress could also be another factor.

Do you get a burning sensation in your stomach?

Clients should not get a burning sensation in their stomachs. Ask how often and if it is after a particular meal. An evening or main meal for example usually contains protein and if the client is deficient in hydrochloric acid, would find it difficult to break down the protein which may result in experiencing the burning sensation. If they get the pain after the main meal, but not with a cereal type breakfast or a smaller meal, this could be the reason. Another good indicator is that the clients feel less pain after a stir-fry type of meal. This is because the protein is already cut up into quite small pieces, hence assisting the digestive system in the early stages of breakdown. Digestive enzymes may assist here. You can purchase Hydrochloric Acid supplementation on its own but I would suggest a digestive enzyme 'multi', containing amylases, proteases, and lipases

Are you prone to stomach upsets?

The first thing I clarify here it the client knows where the stomach is! I point to my abdomen and then to my stomach and ask them where they get their upsets. It is invariably in the abdomen area. Upsets in the abdomen area could be caused by allergies, candida, parasites, or just by eating too much.

Do you use any type of butter or margarine on a daily basis?

A general digestive system question. Most people will answer yes. Advise that butter is better than margarine – just. All butters and margarines hard at room temperature are hydrogenated fats – trans fats – that compromise the body from using other fats effectively. Suggest they use olive oil directly on bread – try it yourself – it tastes good and is a much better source of fat. Alternatively nut butters are a good alternative to ordinary butter. Occasionally is OK but all clients should be encouraged to cut back on saturated fats.

Do you eat quickly/rush your food/eat under stress?

Another common fact of life. Many people just eat too quickly and compromise the whole digestive system which could result in many unpleasant symptoms later. Encourage clients to slow down when food is concerned. Make food and eating times a priority not something that is fitted in-between other events.

Do you normally eat at irregular times?

Not good news. This may lead to a disordered eating pattern which in turn could lead to other problems later. Read the paragraph on 'timing' earlier in this chapter.

ENDOCRINE SYSTEM

Are you taking or have you ever taken the Pill and/or HRT?

The Pill and HRT are both synthetic hormones. One in every 200 women's periods will cease after stopping the Pill and it could take up to two years before fertility will return. Surveys report that 70% of women discontinue HRT within one year and only 7% last eight years.[122] and there are numerous trials showing that HRT significantly increases the risk of breast cancer.

Have you ever had a miscarriage

Around one in four pregnancies are estimated to end in a miscarriage and the real figure is likely to be higher, as many miscarriages go unreported. Some experts believe that miscarriage is a sensitive indicator that the parents are exposed to environmental hazards. One study found that the mother drinking alcohol daily, even in moderation, increased the risk of miscarriage[123]

Do you suffer with any PMS symptoms?

There are many factors associated with PMS but symptoms can be improved by reducing or better still avoiding alcohol, supplementing B6 and zinc one week before a period, reducing stress, and eating large amounts of green leafy vegetables for the magnesium content. There are many different types of PMS symptoms, these are general recommendations.

Do you have difficulty in losing weight?

Many women have difficulty in losing weight. Many just find it difficult to stay on a diet for many reasons. However, if your client is over 45, she may be what is known as 'oestrogen dominant'. In which case one of the main symptoms is difficulty in losing weight. This is a very complex area but a very common one. A natural progesterone cream has proved very helpful for many women approaching the menopause. Investigate progesterone creams and advise clients accordingly.

Do you suffer from lumpy breasts?

Breast tenderness and swelling are symptoms associated with oestrogen dominance and one of 150 different symptoms associated with PMS. Follow the general recommendations for PMS in Part II of this book

Do you suffer from breast tenderness?

As above, associated with oestrogen dominance and therefore progesterone deficiency. Give clients information of progesterone cream.(Appendix I) You are not advising them to use this cream, but you are providing the information so your clients can make informed choices.

Do you often feel tired during the day?

This is one symptom of glucose imbalance. Note what they eat for breakfast and lunch. Is the client eating any protein in these two meals? If no, then by simply adding some protein say an egg for breakfast may make all the difference.

Do you do 2 – 3 tasks simultaneously?

An 'adrenals' question. A 'yes' answer is a sign of anxiety and stress and giving the adrenal glands a hard time. An adrenal support supplement may be recommended or 'time management' skills. Remember the saying 'less haste, more speed'.

Do you have thinning hair on your scalp?

Possible hormone imbalance. Nutri-Hair is an excellent supplement, which could be tried for 6 months – again recommendation to a Nutritional Therapist for hormone testing is recommended. Worry and Stress could make the situation worse so yoga or any stress releasing activity is recommended.

LYMPHATIC SYSTEM AND IMMUNE SYSTEM

Is there a history of cancer in your family?

For clients with a history of cancer in their family, it is even more important to look after themselves. An anti-oxidant is the first recommendation plus all the dietary advice given in the relevant sections of this book.

Do you find it hard to shift an infection?

An indication of a compromised immune system. The healthiest of people get colds from time to time but if the immune system is strong the infection doesn't last long. Vitamin C is a must throughout the winter months. Build up slowly to 1g daily.

Do you sit still for several hours each day? work/TV?

The lymphatic system does not have a heart to act as a pump like the circulatory system. It relies on movement. Contracting muscles through any kind of movement moves lymph along the lymphatic vessels. Sitting for long periods is therefore not recommended for good lymphatics.

Do you avoid physical exercise?

Exercise is important not just for keeping fit or losing weight, but for support for the immune system. Regular movement is needed to keep the lymphatic fluid moving through the vessels to filter toxins for their removal from the body. Avoiding physical exercise will result in an accumulation of toxins in the body.

Do you have cellulite?

Not just for the overweight. I have seen many very slim girls with cellulite. This is a clogging up of the body cells giving the dimpled appearance of the skin. Cellulite does exist and it can be improved. Read up on the cellulite paragraph in the book and advise clients accordingly.

Do you work harder than most people?

This is a 'stress' question and there are many recommendations for a yes answer. Why is your client working harder than most people, could it be an emotional issue? a financial issue? if they constantly need to achieve why is this? Another huge area but immediate help can be given by clients reducing stimulants, taking a daily multi-vitamin and maybe talking to someone if there are any underlying problems.

Do you feel guilty when relaxing?

Another 'stress' question and recommendations as above. Clients may need to 'learn' to relax.

Do you have a persistent need for achievement?

Stress yet again. What drives these people, and why? Probably not in your range of services but to be able to recommend someone if that field is great advice. Think about taking some counselling qualifications yourself — therapists are very often put in a position where some counselling training could come in very useful.

Are you especially competitive?

Stress as above. Continual and persistent stress and competitive events may result in adrenal exhaustion — burnout. A competitive streak is not necessarily bad, but it is important to be nutritionally nourished for any type of competition, be it work or sport related. A daily multi-vitamin is a must for clients in this situation.

Have you taken antibiotics over the past 2 years?

Frequent use of antibiotics suppresses the immune system. Advise clients to always follow up antibiotics with probiotics. Also especially important for children who have had antibiotics — you can purchase special children's formulas of probiotics.

NERVOUS SYSTEM
(scores 2 marks each)

Do you suffer from any type of headache?
Diet can play an important part regarding headaches. It may be that the client is consuming too much of one type of food such as wheat, cheese, or other type of dairy food and may have an intolerance to this food resulting in headaches.

Do you suffer with migraine headaches?
Migraine can be triggered by allergies and may be relieved by identifying and avoiding the problem foods

Do you suffer with 'panic attacks'?
Panic attacks are often the result of excessive anxiety and/or stress. Diet is important in situations involving anxiety and stress. Immediate advice to reduce stress levels, take up yoga, meditation or visualisation. Avoid all junk food and concentrate on eating a really healthy diet of whole foods.

Do you often find yourself irritable/jumpy?
Anti-anxiety and general calming effects on the nervous system have been observed from taking Black Cohosh. Could be related to PMS – needs to be checked. This could also be a symptom of low blood sugar levels/hypoglycemia. Ask what the client does to reduce stress levels. What does she/he understand about stress. It is important to take up relaxing activities like walking, yoga, and meditation.

Do you feel that you lose your temper easily?
Again, could be a symptom of low blood sugar levels, PMS, or excessive stress and anxiety. A calming herb should be recommended and a good look at the diet.

RESPIRATORY SYSTEM

Do you suffer from frequent bronchitis, asthma, colds & flu?
Frequent bouts of the above would suggest that the immune system was compromised and a good multivitamin and mineral would be recommended together with other ways of supporting the immune system.

Do you smoke more than 5 cigarettes per day?
The research shows without any doubt that smoking is dangerous to health, especially in relation to the respiratory system. Every encouragement should be given to your clients to make this a priority task in their life – they won't regret it.

Do you live/work in a smoky atmosphere?

This can be almost as bad as smoking yourself. The smoke breathed out from other people's cigarettes is called cadmium, as is poisonous to us. Encouragement should be given for partners to give up or to at least smoke outside.

Do you (or have you) live/work in a 'chemical' atmosphere? (paint, thinners, petrol, fertilisers, hair sprays, colours etc)

Even with a strong immune system, toxic sprays, the fumes from paints, airborne pollutants all reach the throat and lungs quickly and may result in respiratory problems. A definite need for vitamin C here as with all 'pollution' questions. At least 1g every day is recommended.

Do you eat your fruit and vegetables without washing them?

Unwashed fruit and vegetables are covered with pesticides and could have an immediate effect on your respiratory system. Continued eating of such foods can result in wheezing. Wash everything well, especially around the stalks where pesticides accumulate.

SKELETAL SYSTEM

Do you consume more than 1 pint of milk a day?

It is very important to keep calcium levels up. What you eat during your childhood and teenage years may make all the difference when you are older regarding osteoporosis. Whatever your age, check you are getting enough calcium. Do not forget it comes in green leafy vegetables as well as the dairy produce. However, milk is not a very balanced food — the calcium to magnesium ratio is very poor making it an acidic food. The more acid we have in the diet, the more acidic the system becomes and the more calcium is taken from the bones!! making drinking milk counterproductive. A good balance is ½ a pint of skimmed milk and a small pot of bio-yoghurt per day.

Do you avoid weight-bearing exercise?

Whilst all exercise is important, it is the weight bearing exercise that will keep our bones in good condition. Swimming and cycling, whilst wonderful types of exercise are not weight bearing. Walking, running, playing squash are all weight bearing. No matter how little, every encouragement should be given for clients to do some weight bearing exercise every single day.

Do you eat less than 5 portions of green leafy vegetables and fruit on a daily basis?

A vital component of being healthy is to have at least 5 portions of vegetables and fruit daily. It is the vegetables that will provide the essential minerals needed for health and vitality. If you eat less than the recommended 5 a day then a multivitamin and mineral is strongly recommended.

Do you eat sweet, sugary foods on most days?

A yes answer is not good. Foods like this rob our bodies of vital nutrients. There may be an underlying blood sugar imbalance to look out for. Some clients say they are 'addicted' to sweet foods – which is another indicator of a blood sugar problem.

Do you suffer with any type of arthritis?

Arthritis is an inflammatory condition in the body. One cause can be too much refined foods, red meat, a diet high in saturated fats and sugars. These items make series II prostaglandins in the body which are inflammatory. Your clients need anti-inflammatory foods and supplements. Green vegetables and fruit and lots of oily fish, plus a good supplement regime.

URINARY/ DETOX SYSTEM
Do you suffer with fluid retention?

Fluid retention is a complex subject and not one that should be overlooked. Clients usually need to drink more fluid themselves as the first course of action, and gentle regular daily exercise is always helpful. It is a sign that the body is not eliminating efficiently. Diuretics should be natural ones of which there are many. Watercress, celery, and all the fruits and vegetables.

Have you ever suffered with thrush or cystitis?

Cystitis is a urinary tract infection, which would suggest a compromised immune system. Thrush is a fungal infection sometimes the result of antibiotic use and one of the symptoms of candida albicans. Cranberry Juice and garlic as the first immediate action followed by a full consultation from a nutritional therapist.

Do you suffer from chronic fatigue?

Many reasons for this, but often low blood sugars are one cause. Especially if the clients feel very tired after lunch. An under active thyroid is sometimes also involved. A serious look at the diet should be made with a full client history. Daily supplements of a multivitamin and mineral would be recommended and a visit to a nutritional therapist.

Do you have more than 2 alcoholic drinks a day?

One glass of red wine is reported to be beneficial for the cardiovascular system. Two glasses could be harmful. There are reports and studies showing a case for and against. Alcohol is nutritionally void and often contains only empty calories. If client had candida then alcohol would have to be strictly avoided. Keep alcohol for special occasions and then limit it.

Do you suffer with eczema or psoriasis?

This would again indicate a compromised detoxification system where the kidneys and liver were not working efficiently and the toxins in the body were being released by the skin — also an organ of detoxification. A liver cleanse could be recommended here, or herbal remedies to support the liver. Plenty of water, and the purest, cleanest food obtainable.

Do you suffer from acne or poor skin condition?

Often a sign of zinc deficiency, especially in puberty, where the zinc is being used to mature the reproductive system resulting in the skin suffering. Again, plenty of water, a zinc supplement. Vitamin A is also recommended for skin conditions, plus lots of fresh air and exercise.

Do you feel you have a sensitivity to chemicals?

Many respiratory complaints are the result of airborne substances we have become sensitive to. Perfumes, paints, pollens, yeasts, new carpets can all cause problems. An allergy specialist may be able to pinpoint substances and there are homeopathic remedies to become desensitised to the offending substance.

Do you have any unexplained itching?

Unexplained itching could be many things. Allergy springs to mind and also the skin trying to detoxify the body if the kidneys and liver become sluggish.

Do you drink less than 1 litre of water every day?

Bad news if the answer is yes. This is probably the most important thing we can do for good general health. Really encourage your clients to take up water. Do it yourself too and see the difference. Remember to practice what you preach!

Do you suffer with dull headaches?

Dull headaches could be a sign of dehydration, allergy or stress. Lots of water, rest and every emphasis on relaxation.

MUSCULAR/ENERGY SYSTEM

Is your energy less now than it used to be?

Energy levels need not drop as we get older. If your energy is less now that it used to be it could be a symptom of low blood sugar levels. Too high a carbohydrate diet, a vegetarian diet for example, without sufficient protein and fats to balance is often the cause for energy slumps and feeling tired and lethargic.

Do you avoid exercise due to tiredness?

This is a typical low blood sugar level question. Many clients would love to exercise but just do not have the energy. By changing what they eat and quite often when they eat, energy levels can be restored and exercise can resume. Small frequent meals containing carbohydrates, proteins and essential fatty acids at each meal and snack time, can change the body's chemical activity so much, the client will be running to the gym!

Do you sweat a lot or get excessively thirsty?

Diabetics get excessively thirsty and thirst is one of the symptoms that build up over the years in clients who handle sugar badly. It is called the Glucose Tolerance Factor and unless it is kept in check, could result insulin resistance or even diabetes much in later life. Sweating without exercise is also another symptom in the Glucose Tolerance Factor.

Do you get dizzy or irritable if you don't eat often?

A typical reaction for people with low blood sugar. Eating little and often is the first course of action. Each meal or snack should include complex carbohydrate, protein and essential fatty acids. The protein and fat will slow down the release of sugar in the body.

Do you often feel drowsy during the day

Still on the same subject of Glucose Tolerance Factor. If 'yes' then more protein, less carbohydrate may be necessary for particular clients. A jacket potato and beans for lunch could have a client falling asleep at the desk, whereas a jacket potato with tuna plus a mixed salad with a trickle of olive oil would probably have an entirely different effect.

Do you sometimes lose concentration?

A sign that the brain is not receiving glucose. Eating little and often may help the situation, and again, if breakfast and/or lunch is a carbohydrate only affair, then give suggestions of adding a little protein and essential fatty acids (nuts, seeds, olives, avocado) not saturated fats.

Do you suffer with cramps?
Usually a magnesium deficiency as one of the functions of magnesium is to relax the muscles. Check with the client how much green leafy vegetables they are eating. Encourage to eat more, or suggest a calcium:magnesium supplement.

Do you suffer with muscular aches and pains?
No matter what age your client, suffering with aches and pains is something that can be overcome. Green leafy vegetables are full of magnesium and are of immense benefit for muscles. The supplement MSM (organic sulphur) is excellent for aches and pains and comes highly recommended. Gentle exercise, although the last thing they probably want to do is also a great remedy and very effective. Also investigate food allergy.

Do you have much injury through playing sport?
All body systems need supporting. Good multivitamins and minerals and plenty of water. Most athletes need more supplementation than average as they are working hard at their sport. The diet needs working on or injury will occur through dehydration and malnutrition. People can be fit without being healthy, and look good on the outside while weak on the inside. MSM another good supplement for athletes and Chromium.

Do you drink less than 8 glasses of water every day?
Muscles need water. So many symptoms can be put down to dehydration. The energy system of the body needs water (not in tea or coffee and not carbonated) just plain bottled spring water. This will reduce injury and hydrate.

SUPPLEMENTARY QUESTIONS

Here are some additional questions you may like to ask your client, with explanations of the answers – they are not in any particular order and some may appear similar to some of the questions above.

Do you go out of your way to avoid sweet, sugary, foods?
The answer to this should be 'yes'. If the answer is 'no' then you should be giving encouragement to your client that sweet, sugary foods upset the delicate blood sugar balance in the body, as well as containing little or no nutrients. Quality should be a key word when selecting food.

Do you drink 6 – 8 glasses of water *every day?*

One of the most important aspects of good nutrition is to have 6–8 glasses of water every day. The human body is 70% water and we need it to flush the system taking toxic substances with it. Essential for a clear, healthy skin.

Do you normally eat at regular times?

Unfortunately, many people do not. Read the paragraph on timing and ask the client to do the exercise in writing down the times they are going to eat their food. This one small change in their life could make so much difference to how they feel.

Do you have a bowel movement every day?

The answer to this should be yes, but being 'regular' to some people may be every other day, which is fine. However, they should work on going at least once a day.

How much water do you drink in one day. Is this bottled water or tap water?

This is a 'chemical' type question. Bottled water is better, tap water may contain harmful additives that are building up inside your client that may result in internal pollution. The answer should be 6 – 8 glasses a day. If it is less than this then the body may become dehydrated and hold- on to water resulting in dehydration.

Salt intake. Do you add salt to your cooking and/or add it to your food?

This is a cardiovascular question. The more salt a client has in the diet, the higher risk of cardiovascular disease. If your answer is 'yes' to either of these statements your recommendation would be to cut down on at least one or better still both methods of adding salt.

How much sugar do you add to your diet daily in tea/coffee/on cereals/in food.?

The more sugar in the diet, the more refined it probably is and will give rise to weight gain, unbalanced blood sugar balance in the body. Sugar has no nutrients – there are much better ways to make food sweet.

How many pints of milk do you drink in a week?

A general nutrition question regarding calcium. Obtaining enough calcium (800mg for adults) is essential for healthy bones and teeth and for the prevention of osteoporosis. Your recommendations will depend upon the answer you are given. You must stress the importance of calcium and give other sources for the client's information.

How many times a week do you eat red meat?

Another general nutrition question. Whilst red meat provides important protein, it is also a source of saturated fat and could contain traces of antibiotics or growth hormones, which would be undesirable. 3 times a week would be maximum and encouragement to eat a less fat source of protein like chicken, turkey, or fish.

Do you eat at regular times?

An important question. Many people eat at irregular times. Sometimes when you eat is more important than what you eat. Regulating eating times is the first step in good weight management. Breakfast is, of course, the most important meal and every encouragement should be given to clients to eat a healthy breakfast. Without breakfast, blood sugar levels may be low and clients may be 'running on empty' to get to work/school. If the first thing they have is coffee/tea/biscuits then this will push blood sugar levels up and this pattern of rising and falling could continue throughout the day.

Are you vegetarian/vegan

If the answer is 'yes' – you need to ensure that the client is receiving sufficient calcium and protein from their diet. Many clients, especially teenagers, are unaware of the importance of these nutrients for normal body and brain development. Daily servings of chips and crisps may well be vegetarian but will also lead to malnutrition.

Do you suffer from fluid retention?

If the answer is yes, first of all ascertain whether it is cyclic. If yes then it is more than likely involved with the hormonal response to the monthly cycle. If no, then ask if client is on medication. Many medications for blood pressure, anxiety, migraines, have side effects of fluid retention and/or weight gain. Check if the fluid retention started about the same time as the medication. Ask the client to discuss with her GP if they think the medication could be a cause. Advise client of some of the many natural diuretics available to them.

Which foods would you find hard to give up?

It is highly likely that the foods a client will include in this section may well be foods that they are sensitive to. Wheat is a common answer. Encourage clients to eat wheat only 2 or 3 times a week. Study their 3–day food plan. Are they eating wheat 3 times a day? eg Weetabix for breakfast, a sandwich for lunch followed by pasta for dinner? This is very common and should be discouraged. Always give alternatives. In this case encourage rice, quinoa, corn, barley, or rye.

Do you ever experience joint pains?

If 'yes' then this could be connected to allergy, candida or hormonal imbalances. Further questions would be necessary. Recommend MSM (organic sulphur) and/or glucosamine sulphate.

Do you suffer from food cravings?

Another multi-faceted question. If yes, they could be connected with allergy, glucose intolerance or candida. Further investigations are needed.

Do you especially crave foods pre-menstrually?

Unlike the question above, these food cravings are hormonally based.

Do you live in a city or busy road?

If 'yes' then this client would probably be breathing in excessive car fumes, which are 'anti nutrients' and would be having a detrimental effect on their health generally. Vitamin C is recommended for any type of 'pollution' problem.

Do you live or work in a smoky atmosphere?

Another 'pollution' question. Cadmium – the substance breathed out by smokers, is just as detrimental to your health as nicotine. Vitamin C is the recommended nutrient.

Do you have athlete's foot, ringworm, 'jock itch' or other chronic fungal infections of the skin or nails?

If 'yes' this may be one indication of a candida infestation. Other questions would need to be asked.

Do your stools float?

The answer should be a 'yes'. Eating a high fibre diet with plenty of fruit and vegetables and sufficient protein and fats, will ensure good bowel function.

Are you trying to become pregnant?

Much can be done from a nutritional point of view for women trying to conceive. Both the male and female should take a zinc supplement on a daily basis as this is a vital mineral in the fertility process. Avoid coffee, tea, alcohol and anything synthetic and enjoy the best possible diet by way of green leafy vegetables, and low fat protein. Maybe a complete lifestyle change for some people — but look at the rewards.

Do you have excess hair on your body?

Possible hormonal imbalance. Recommend your clients sees a Nutritional Therapist who will be able to look into the area more thoroughly and advise if any hormone tests are needed

Do you get more than three colds a year?

If you are prone to colds then Vitamin C is even more important. Take up to bowel tolerance. Everyone has a different level of bowel tolerance of vitamin C, but if the body is saturated with it, then cold viruses cannot survive. Start slowly, and gradually build up increasing a little more each day until the stool becomes quite soft — that will be your level of tolerance. Vitamin C is probably the safest of all the vitamins. At the onset of a cold take 1g and repeat every 4 hours for the first three days. Continue taking at a level you feel is right for you. This could be 2g daily or it could be up to 5g daily. Find out your own tolerance.

Do you often do 2 or 3 tasks simultaneously?

Mental stress, which could result in insomnia. Doing one thing thoroughly, at a time, usually gets more done at the end of the day. Time management needed for clients with a daily achievable 'to do' list.

Do you have eczema, asthma or arthritis?

Very often a deficiency in Essential Fatty Acids. Supplementing EFA's by way of fish oils and Evening Primrose or Starflower oils may have positive results. See separate entries in Part II of this book.

Do you bruise easily?

Easy bruising is a sign of vitamin C deficiency. Vitamin C strengthens capillary walls and makes collagen.

Do you suffer from broken capillaries or thread veins?

Another sign of vitamin C deficiency. Vitamin C strengthens capillary walls.

BODY MASS INDEX

Your Body Mass Index (BMI) gives a good indication of whether you are a healthy weight. To work out your BMI:

1. Work out your height in meters (see the height chart opposite) and multiply the figure by itself.
2. Measure your weight in kilograms
3. Divide the weight (question 2) by the height squared (i.e. the answer to question 1). For example, you might be 1.6m (5 foot 3 inches) tall and weigh 65kg (10 stone). The calculation would then be 1.6 x 1.6 = 2.56. Your BMI would be 65 divided 2.56 = 25.39.

Now work out your BMI and check your result against the table below. But before you do, remember not to take it too seriously! Stocky people (and girls in particular) may appear to be overweight when using this method. So be honest with yourself. If you are naturally of a stocky build do not try to lose weight unnecessarily.

Remember
The BMI is just an **indicator** to ascertain a healthy weight There are other factors to take into account

Category	Range
Underweight	Less than 20
Ideal	20–25
Overweight; advisable to lose weight if you are under 50	25–30
You should lose weight	30–40
Definitely too fat; lose weight now	Greater than 40

HEIGHT CHART

Feet and inches	Meters	Feet and inches	Meters
4′ 10″	1.45	5′ 9″	1.74
4′ 11″	1.5	5′ 10″	1.78
5′	1.52	5′ 11″	1.8
5′ 1″	1.55	6′	1.82
5′ 2″	1.57	6′ 1″	1.85
5′ 3″	1.6	6′ 2″	1.88
5′ 4″	1.62	6′ 3″	1.9
5′ 5″	1.65	6′ 4″	1.92
5′ 6″	1.68	6′ 5″	1.95
5′ 7″	1.7	6′ 6″	1.98
5′ 8″	1.72	6′ 7″	2

If your BMI falls within the ideal range and you are the right weight, that's great, but it is still important to eat healthily to receive all the nutrients needed to stay healthy, fit and well. It is also important not to put on weight. People aged 30 – 74 with BMIs at the lower end of the normal range have the lowest death rates. And people who stay the same weight in middle age as they were in their youth live longer, are generally healthier and therefore more able to enjoy themselves.

HIP TO WAIST RATIO

Whilst the Body Mass Index is a good general indicator of if you are overweight or not, but the hip to waist ratio is probably a better indicator. The risk of heart disease doesn't only depend on how much fat you're carrying, its also where you are carrying it that matters. Our genes determine out basic shape; whether the fat on your body is deposited around our hips, breasts and upper arms (women) so that we are pear-shaped, or whether excess fat is deposited around our abdomens making men and some women apple shaped.

It may seem unfair but if apple shaped people become overweight they are at greater risk of heart disease and diabetes than pear-shaped people.

To make the calculation:-

1. Measure your waist and hips
2. Then divide the waist measurement by the hip measurement to get your waist-hip ratio.

For example, if your waist is 86cm (34 inches) and your hips 102cm (40 inches), your waist-hip ratio will be 86 divided by 102 = 0.85. If the ratio of your waist to hip measurement is more than 0.95 as a man and more than 0.87 as a woman you are apple shaped.

There is another rule of thumb as far as waist measurements are concerned. If a man has a waist that measures more than 94cm (37 inches), or a woman's is more than 80cm (31 inches), they are categorized by some doctors as overweight. Waists do thicken with age, a phenomenon often referred to as 'middle age spread'. If you are younger and already have a 'spare tyre' – act now. It is this abdominal fat that increases the risk of heart disease.

FOOD ENERGY VALUES

A calorie is the amount of energy that is released as heat when food is metabolised. Scientists determine the number of calories in foods by burning them in a laboratory device called a calorimeter and measuring the amount of heat produced. The calorie is the amount of heat necessary to raise the temperature of one liter of water one degree Celsius.

Carbohydrates and protein contain 4 calories per gram whereas fat contains 9 calories per gram, and alcohol 7 calories per gram.

The nutrient content of different foods as compared to their caloric content is the basis of what dietitians call 'nutrient density'. Some foods are naturally healthy to consume, with a high nutrient value in relation to their caloric (energy) content. A fundamental rule of diet planning to promote health is to choose foods with a high nutrient density. Problems arise when needed nutrients are missing from a diet, as well as when too many calories are consumed for daily energy needs. Whole grains and beans provide enough B vitamins to help process the energy they contain, and therefore, are of proper nutrient density. A white flour high-fat food may contain more calories than its nutrient value can handle and this robs health.

Most diets concentrate on ways of eating fewer calories, however in practice calorie restricted diets do not work. I have witnessed many clients that have been on liquid only diets and lost up to four stones in weight. Unfortunately these clients put it all the weight back on again and more whilst some experienced extensive hair loss and others ended up on Prozac because of depression.

Aim at eliminating the word 'diet' from your vocabulary and that of your clients. It is a negative word that stops many people before they even start. Encourage a healthy eating plan – not a plan that will last a few weeks before resuming their normal diet – but a new healthy eating plan that will become their 'normal' diet.

By avoiding the foods that are high in saturated fats, refined sugars and alcohol, and replacing with whole foods, fruit and vegetables, then weight loss will be inevitable.

CONTRAINDICATIONS FOR NUTRITIONAL ADVICE

If you are not already suitably qualified in nutrition, the following are a list of contraindications should be adhered to: Do not offer nutritional advice to the following groups of people, unless you obtain permission from their GP stating otherwise.

Clients under 18 or over 70 years of age.
Clients currently undergoing medical treatment.
Clients with severe obesity.
Clients suffering with an eating disorder.
Clients who have a medically identified food intolerance.
Clients already on a medically prescribed diet.
Clients who are severely underweight.
Clients who are pregnant.

HOW MUCH HAVE YOU REMEMBERED?

SELF-TEST No 1 — CARBOHYDRATES

1. What is the main function of carbohydrates?
2. What is the main difference between mono-saccahrides and polysaccharides?
3. Give 5 reasons why fibre is important in the diet
4. What are enzymes?
5. Name the enzyme needed for the breakdown of carbohydrates in the body.

SELF-TEST No 2 — PROTEINS

1. How many essential amino acids are there?
2. What are the main functions of protein?
3. What is a 'limiting' amino acid?
4. What 4 particular nutrients are needed by the liver to convert the essential amino acids to other amino acids?
5. Which particular essential amino acid is often low in vegetarian diets and what foods can this be found in?

SELF-TEST No 3 — FATS

1. What are the three main divisions of fats?
2. What are the main functions of fats?
3. What are prostaglandins?
4. How can fibre help lower cholesterol levels?
6. What are Series 2 prostaglandins?

SELF-TEST No 4 — SUPPLEMENTS

1. Vitamins are divided into two main divisions. What are they?
2. What do the initials SONA stand for and when should we use them?
3. An excess of copper in the body may result in a deficiency of which mineral?
4. What is Co-Q-10 and what is its function?
5. What are the antioxidants, and what is their main function?

SELF-TEST No 5 — HERBS

Q1 What is the main function of herbs?

Q2 Which herb has anti-histamine, antioxidant and anti-inflammatory properties and is usually recommended for allergies?

Q3 Which herb has anti-depressant, anti-bacterial, and sedative properties and is usually recommended for mild depression?

Q4 What important difference must you remember between the herbs Vitex (Agnus Castus) and Black Cohosh?

Q5 If a client had poor circulation, especially to their hands and feet, what herb might you consider?

SELF-TEST No 6 — SUPERFOODS

1. What superfood would you consider for a vegan or strict vegetarian?

2. Honey can be described as a prebiotic. What are prebiotics, and what other foods come into this category?

3. Which superfood is anti-bacterial, anti-viral, and heals stomach ulcers?

4. Which of the superfoods his anti-viral properties, and benefits respiratory tract infections?

5. What are the main functions of Bee Pollen?

6. Unlike blue-green algae, spirulina and chlorophyll, mushrooms lack chlorophyll. Where do these medicinal mushrooms obtain their healing properties?

(Answers can be found in Appendix 2)

REFERENCES

1. Bradley PR, ed. *British Herbal Compendium*, vol. 1. Bournemouth, Dorset, UK: British Herbal Medicine Association, 1992, 112–4

2. Yamahara J, Huang Q, et al. *Gastro intestinal motility enhancing effect of ginger and its active constituents. Chem Pharm Bull* 1990;38:430–1

3. Al-Yahta MA, Rafatullah S, et al. *Gastro protective activity of ginger in albino rats. Am J Chinese Med* 1989;17:51–6

4. Holtman S, Clarke AH, et al. *The anti-motion sickness mechanism of ginger. Acta Otolaryngol (Stockh)* 1989;108: 168–74.

5. Suekawa M, Isgige A, et al. *Pharmacological studies on ginger. I. Pharmacological actions of pungent constituents* (6)-gingerol and (6)-shogaol. *J Pharm Dyn* 1984;7:836–48

6. Bone ME, Wilkinson DJ, Young JR, et al. *Ginger root – a new antiemetic: The effect of ginger root on postoperative nausea and vomiting after major gynacological surgery. Anaesthesia* 1990; 45:669–71

7. Phillips S, Ruggier R, Hutchingson SE. *Zingiber officinale* (ginger) – an antiemetic for day case surgery. *Anaesthesia* 1993;48:715–7

8. Grontved A, Brask T, Kambskard J, Hentzer E. *Ginger root against seasickness. Acta Otolaryngo 1* 1988;105:45–9

9. Ribenfeld D, Borzone L. *Randomised double-blind study comparing ginger (Zintona®) with dimengydrinate in motion sickness. Healthnotes Rev Complementary Intergrative Med* 1999;6:98–101

10. Careddu P. *Motion sickness in children: Results of a double blind study comparing ginger (Zintona®) and dimenhydrinate. Healthnotes Rev Complementary Intregratrive Med* 1999;6:102–7

11. Meyer K, Schwartz J, Craer D, Keyes B. *Zinger officinale (ginger) used to prevent 8–Mop associated nausea. Dermatol Nursing* 1995;7:242–4

12. Langner E, Greifenberg S, Gruenwald J. *Ginger: History and use. Adv Ther* 1998;15:25–44 (review)

13. Brunner, R., Tabaehnik, B. (1990) *Soviet Training and Recovery Methods,* pp217–21. Sport Focus Publishing

14. Cheraskin, E et al., '*Establishing a suggested optimum nutrition allowance (SONA)*', 1994

15. Luce A *Amazing Micro-Algae* Optimum Nutrition Volume 12:3 Autumn 1999

16. Chang, R., *Functional properties of edible mushrooms*' Nutr Rev (1996), 54(11 Pt2):S91–93

17. Ishigami, H., et al., *Relationship between prolonged life span and changes of serum LAP and albumin induced by the therapy of lentinan plus tegafur in inoperable and recurrent gastric cancer*' Nippon Geka Gakkai Zasshi (1992) 93:800–04.

18. Levy, A.M., et al., *Eosinophilia and gastrointestinal symptoms after ingestion of shiitake mushrooms*' J Allergy clin Immunol (1998), 101 (5):613–20

19. Luckes M., *Health from the Hive* Optimum Nutrition Volume 13:2 Spring 2000

20. Carper Jean *Food Your Miracle Medicine* The Amazing Cabbage Experiments p217.

21. Firshein R Dr. *the Nutraceutical Revolution*' Vermilion Books p.97

22. Mohr H, *Clinical Investigations of means to increase lactation,* Dtsch Med Wschr 1954;79(41):1513–6

23. Weiss, R.R. *Herbal Medicine* Ab Arctum, Stockholm, Sweden, 1988

24. Peters-Welte, C and Albrecht, M: *Menstrual abnormalities and PMS:* Vitex agnus-castus. TW Gynekologie 7:49–52,1994

25. Mennini T, Bernasconi P, et al. *In vitro study on the interaction of extracts and pure compo from Valeriana officinalis roots with GABA, benzodiazepine and barbiturate receptors.* Fitote 1993;64:291–300

26. Kohnen R, Oswald WD. *The effects of valerian, propranolol and their combination on active performance and mood of healthy volunteers under social stress conditions.* Pharmacop. 1988;21:447–48

27. Leathwood PD, Chauffard F, Heck E, Munoz-Box R. *Aqueous extract of valerian root (Vale officinalis L) improves sleep quality in man. Pharmacol Biochem Behav* 1982;17:65–71

28. Leathwood PD, Chauffard F, *Aqueous extract of valerian reduces latency to fall asleep* Planta Med 1985;51:144–148

29. Lindahl O, Lindwall L. *double blind study of a valerian preparation.* Pharmacol Biochem 1989;32:1065–66

30. Hepato-Gastroentrology 26:257–259, 1979

31. American Journal of clinical Nutrition 32:1898–1901,1979

32. British Medical Journal, September 29, 1929

33. Digestion 20:323–326, 1980

34. British Medical Journal, April 9, 1977, page 929

35. Passmore AP, Wilson-Davies K, et al. *Chronic constipation in long stay elderly patients: A comparison of lactulose and senna-fiber combination* BMJ 1993; 307:769–71

36. James JM, Burks AW. *Food-associated gastrointestinal disease.* Curr Opin Pediatr 1996; 75 (review).

37. Haffejee IE. *Effect of oral folate on duration of acute infantile diarrhoea.* Lancet 1988,ii:33(letter)

38. Babb RR. *Coffee, sugars and chronic diarrhea.* Prostgrad Med 1984;75:82,86–87

39. Werbach MR. *Nutritional Influences on Illness* 2ed Tarzana, CA Third Line press, 256–61 (review)

40. Bhan J, Bhandari N. *The role of zinc and vitamin A in persistent diarrhoea among infants and young children.* J Pediatr Gastroenterol Nutri 1998;26:446–53 (review)

41. Hyams JS, Etienne NL, Leichtner AM, Theuer RC. *Carbohydrate malabsorption following fructose ingestion in young children.* Pediatr 1988; 82:64–68.

42. Barness LA. *Safety considerations with high ascorbic acid dosage.* Ann NY Acad Sci 1975; 258:523–28 (review).

43. Achterrath-Tuckerman U, Kunde R, etal. *pharmacological investigations with compounds of chamomile. V. Investigations on the spasmolytic effect of compounds of chamomile on isolated guinea pig ileum.* Planta Med 1980; 39:38–50.

44. Schulz V, Hansel R, Tyler VE. *Rational Phytotherapy: A Physician's Guide to Herbal Medicine.* 3rd ed. Berlin. Springer, 1998, 168–73

45. Murray MJ, Stein N. *A gastric factor promoting iron absorption.* Lancet 1968; 1:614

46. Ivanovich P et al. *The absorption of calcium carbonate.* Ann Intem Med 1967;66:917

47. Recker RR. *Calcium absorption and achlorhydria.* JEJM 1985; 313:70

48. Sturdiolo GC et al. *Inhibition of gastric acid secretion reduces zinc absorption in man.* J AM Nutr 1991; 10:372–75

49.   Allison JR. *The relation of hydrochloric acid and vitamin B complex deficiency in certain skin conditions* South Med J 1945; 38:235

50.   Russell RM et al. *Correction of impaired folic acid (Pte Glu) absorption by orally administered in subjects with gastric atrophy.* AM J Clin Nutr 1984; 39:656

51.   Mayron LW. *Portals of entry*: A review. Ann Allergy 1978; 40:399

52.   Walker WA, Isselbacher KJ. *Uptake and transport of macro-molecules by the intestine. Positive role in clinical disorder.* Gastroenterology 1974; 67:531

53.   Gastroenterology 1969; 56(1):71ff.

54.   Giannella RA. *Influence of gastric acidity on bacterial and parasitic enteric infections.* A perspective. Ann Int Med 1973; 78:271–76

55.   Kraft K. *Artichoke leaf extract – recent findings reflecting effects on lipid metabolism, liver and gastrointestinal tracts.* Phytomedicine 1997; 4:370–78 review.

56.   Kirchhoff R, Beckers C, Kirchhoff GM, et al. *Increase in choleresis by means of artichoke extract* Phytomedicine 1994;1:107–15

57.   Cann, P.A.Read, N.W., Holdsworth, C.D. What is the benefit of coarse wheat bran in patients with irritable bowel syndrome? Gut 1984; 25:168–173

58.   Arfmann, S., Andersen, J.R., Hegnhoj, J. et al. irritable bowel syndrome treated with wheat bran – a controlled double blind trial. Scand J Gastroenterol 1983; 18(S86)3.

59.   Gaby, A.R. Commentary. Nutrition and Healing, Feb 1996: 1,10–11 (review)

60.   Houghton, L.A., Heyman, D., Whorwell, P.J. Hypnotherapy: effect on quality of life and economic consequences of irritable bowel syndrome. Gut 1994; 35 (suppl 5) abstract # F231.

61.   Cotterell, C.J., Lee, A.J., Hunter, J.O. *double blind cross-over trial of evening primrose oil in women with menstrually-related irritable bowel syndrome. In Omega-6 Essential Fatty Acids:* Pathophysiology and roles in clinical medicine, Alan R. Liss, New York, 1990; 421–426

62.   Dew, M.J, Evans, B.K. Rhodes, J. *Peppermint oil for the irritable bowel syndrome: A multi-centre trial.* Br. J. Clin Pract 1984; 38:394–398

63.   Achterrath-Tuckerman, U., Kunde, R., et al. *Pharmacological investigations with compounds of chamomile V. Investigations on the spasmolytic effect of compounds of chamomile and Kamillosan on isolated guinea pig ileum.* Planta Med 1980; 39:38–50

64.   Westphal, J., Horning, M., Leonhardt, K. *Phytotherapy in functional abdominal complaints: Results of a clinical study with a preparation of several plants.* Phytomed 1996; 2:285–291.

65.   Allison MC, Howatson AG, Caroline MG, et al. *Gastrointestinal damage associated with the use of non-steroidal anti-inflammatory drugs.* N Engl J Med 1992; 327:749–54

66.   Lenz HJ, Ferrari-Taylor J, Isenberg JJI. *Wine and five per cent ethanol are potent stimulants in gastric acid secretion in humans.* Gastroenterology 1983; 85:1082–87

67.   Cohen S, Booth GH Jr. *Gastric acid secretion and lower-esophageal-spincter pressure in response to coffee and caffeine.* N Engl J Med 1975; 293:897–99

68.   Feldman EJ, Isenberg JI, Grossman MI. *Gastric acid and gastrin response to decaffeinated coffee and a peptone meal.* JAMA 1981; 246:248–50

69.   Dubey P, Sundram KR, Nundy S. *Effect of tea on gastric acid secretion.* Dig Dis Sci 1984; 29:202–6

70. Korman MG, Hansky J, Eaves ER, Schmidt GT. *Influence of cigarette smoking onhealing relapse in duodenal ulcer disease*. Gastroenterology 1983; 85:871–74

71. Cheney G. *Rapid healing of peptic ulcers in patients receiving fresh cabbage juice*. Cal Med 1949; 70:10

72. Doll R, Pygott F. *Clinical trial of Robaden and of cabbage juice in the treatment of gastric ulcers* Lancet 1954; ii:1200

73. Thaly H. *A new therapy of peptic ulcer. The anti-ulcer factor of cabbage*. Gaz Med Fr 1965; 72:1992–93

74. Dunaevskii GA, Migonova DK, Rozka IM, Chibisova SM. *Value of preserved juice of white cabbage in the complex therapy of peptic ulcer*. Vopr Pital 1970; 29:29–33

75. Noess K. *Ulcer-fiber-cabbage and vitamin U*. Tidsskr Nor Laegeforen 1986; 106:693–94

76. Kern RA, Stewart G. *Allergy in duodenal ulcer: incidence and significance of food hypersensitivities as observed in 32 patients*. J Allergy 1931; 3:51

77. Reiman HJ, Lewin J. Gastric mucosal reactions in patients with food allergy. Am J Gastr 1988; 83:1212–19

78. Sivam GP, Lampe JW, Ulness B, et al. *Helicobacter pylori – in vitro susceptibility to garlic (Allium sativum) extract* Nutr Cancer 1997; 27:118–21

79. Tabak M, Armon R, Potasman I, Neeman I *In vitro inhibition of Heliocobacter pylori by extract of thyme* J Appl Bacteriol 1996; 80 (6):667–72

80. Deanfield J, Wright C, Krikler S,et al. *Cigarette smoking and the treatment of angina with propranolol, atenolol, and nifedipine*. N Engl J Med 1984; 310:951–54

81. Cherchi A, Lai C, Angelino F, et al. *Effects of L-carnitine on exercise tolerance in chronic stage angina: A multicenter, double-blind, randomised, placebo-controlled crossover study*. Int J Clin Pharm Ther Toxicol 1985; 23:569–72

82. Canale C, Terrachini V, Biagini A, et al. *Bicycle ergometer and echocardiographic study in subjects and patients with angina pectoris after administration of L-carnitine in patients with exercise in stable angina*: A controlled study. Drugs Exp Clin Res 1991; 17:225–35.

83. Cacciatore L, Cerio R, et al. The therapeutic effect of L-carnitine in patients with exercise stable angina.

84. Kamikawa T, Kobayashi, A, Yamashita T, et al. *Effects of coenzyme Q10 on exercise tolerance in chronic stable angina pectoris*. Am J Cardiol 1985: 56:247

85. Mortensen SA. *Perspectives on therapy of cardiovascular disease with coenzyme Q10 (ubiquinone)*. Clin Invest 1993; 71:s116–23 (review)

86. Riemersma RA, Wood DA, Macintyre CC, et al. *Risk of angina pectoris and plasma concentrations of vitamins A, C and E and carotene*. Lancet 1991; 337:1–5

87. Rinzler SH, Bakst H, Benjamin ZH, et al. *Failure of alpha-tocopherol to influence chest pain patients with heart disease*. Circulation 1950; 1:288–90

88. Saynor R, Verel D, Gillott T. *The long-term effect of dietary supplementation with fish lipid concentrate on serum lipids, bleeding time, platelets and angina*. Atheroscl 1984; 50:3–10

89. Wander RC, Du SH, Ketchum SO, Rowe KE. *Alpha-tocopherol influences in vivo indices peroxidation in postmenopausal women given fish oil*. J Nutr 1996; 126:643–52

90. Mirelman D, Monheir D, Varon S. Inhibition of growth of Entamoeba histolytica by allicin, the active principle of garlic extract (Allium sativum). *J Infect Dis* 1987;156: 243–44

91. Bastidas CJ. Effect of ingested garlic on Necator americanus and Ancylostoma caninum. *Am J Trop Med Hyg* 1969;13: 920–23

92. Koch HP, Lawson LD, Eds. *Garlic: The Science and Therapeutic Application of Allium sativum L. and Related Species.* Baltimore: Williams & Wilkins, 1996, 173–74

93. Kaplan KH, Goldberg DL, Galvin-Naduea M. *The impact of a meditation-based stress reduction program on fibromyalgia.* Gen Hosp Psychiatry 1993; 15:284–89

94. Sprott H, Frankle S, Hluge H, Hein G. *Pain treatment of fibromyalgia by acupuncture* Rheumatol Int 1998; 18:35–36

95. Wilke W. Fibromyalgia: *Recognizing and addressing the multiple interrelated factors.* Postgrad Med 1996;100(1):153–170

96. Steinberg CL. *The tocopherols (vitamin E) in the treatment of primary fibrositis.* J Bone Joint Surg 1942; 24:411–23

97. Carette S. *Fibromyalgia 20 years later: What have we really accomplished?* J Rheumatol 1995; 22(4):590–94

98. Mengshail AM, Komnaes HB, Forre O. The effects of 20 weeks of physical fitness training in female patients with fibromyalgia. *Clin Exp Rheumatol* 1992;10: 345–49

99. Wright JV *Dr. Wright's Guide to Healing with Nutrition.* New Canaan, CT: Keats Publishing 1990, 155.

100. *'Tomato Lycopene and Low Density Lipoprotein Oxidation: A Human Dietary Intervention Study'* Agarwal S and Rao AV, *Lipids,* 1998; 33(10):981–984 (Address: A Venketeshwer Rao, Department of Nutritional Sciences, Faculty of Medicine, University of Toronto, Toronto, Ontario, M5S 3E2, Canada) 31102

101. *Effects of Pistachio Nuts on Serum Lipid Levels in Patients With Moderate Hypercholesterolemia* Edwards K, et al *J Am Coll Nutr,* 1999; 18(3):229–232

102. *Better Health Through Natural Healing,* Ross Trattler p.317

103. *Better Health Through Natural Healing,* Ross Trattler p.323

104. *Effects of Pistachio Nuts on Serum Lipid Levels in Patients with Moderate Hypercholesterolemia* Edwards K, et al., J Am Coll Nutr, 1999; 18(3): 229–232. (Address Karen Edwards, MS, 11444 West Olympic Blvd, Los Angeles, CA 90064, USA) 32246

105. Coronary Heart Disease and Flavonoids. Nutrition Week, June 4, 1999; 29 (21):7/AM J Epidemiol, May 15, 1999; 149(10): 943–949. 32440A

106. Oxford Concise Medical Dictionary. Ed. E.A. Martin, OUP, 1998

107. The BMA Complete Family Health Encyclopedia. Ed. T. Smith, Dorling, Kindersley 1995

108. Human Nutrition and Dietetics, J Garrow & W James, Churchill Livingstone, 9th edition 1993

109. *New England Journal of Medicine* 1997, 337; 670–6

110. *Nutrition,* 1992; 8: 400–405

111. *Arthritis,* Prof. P A Dieppe, Equation, 1988

112. *British Journal of Rheumatology,* June 1993, 32; 6: 507–14

113. Tortora – *The Principals of the Human Body* page 777.

114. Better Health through Natural Healing, Ross Trattler p.546

114. Barnes, Broda, *Hypothyroidism: The Unsuspected Illness*, Harper & Row, New York, 1976

115. Rose, R: *Endocrine responses to stressful psychological events.* Psych Clin N Amer 3:251–75, 1980

116. Keller, S.E., Weiss, J.M. Schleifer, SJ. et al: *Suppression of immunity by stress: Effects of graded series of stressors on lymphocyte stimulation in the rat.* Science 213:1397, 1981

117. Total Wellness, Joseph Pizzorno, N.D. Chapter 4, page 50

118. Aydin S, Ercan M, Caskurlu T, et al. *Acupuncture and hypnotic suggestions in the treatment of non-organic male sexual dysfunction.* Scand J Urol Nephrol 1997;31:271–74

119. Zorgniotti AW, Lizza EF. *Effect of large doses of the nitric oxide precursor, L-arginine, on erectile dysfunction.* Int J Impot Res 1994;6:33–36

120. Soyka F, Edmonda A *The ION Effect.* New York:Bantam 1977

121. Cohen AJ, Bartlik B. *Ginkgo biloba for antidepressant-induced sexual dysfunction.* J Sex Marital Ther 1998;24:139–43

122. *'Heard the one about the Pill? It's a Killer!' L Carpenter* — Balancing Hormones Naturally, ION Press, K. Neil, 1994

123. *Lancet (26 July 1980)* also in *Good Health Guide,* Bloomsbury Health Publisher

124. Rapola RM, Virtamo J, Haukka JK et al. *Effect of vitamin E and beta carotene on the incidence of angina pectoris.* A randomised, double blind, controlled trial. JAMA 1996; 275:693–98

125. Miwa K, Miyagi Y, Igawa A, et al. *Vitamin E deficiency in variant angina.* Circulation 1996; 94:14–18

126. Tyler V. Herbs of Choice: *The Therapeutic Use of Phytomedicinals.* New York: Pharmace Products Press, 1994, 74 (review).

127. Piller NB. *A comparison of the effectiveness of some anti-inflammatory drugs* Br J Exp Pathol 1975; 56:554–59

128. Becker HM, Niedermaier G, Orend KH, *Benzopyrone in the therapy of post reconstructive A clinical double-blind study.* Fortschr Med 1985; 103:593–96 (in German)

129. Egger J, Carter CM, Wilson J, et al. *Is migraine food allergy?* A double blind controlled trial of oligoantigenic diet treatment. Lancet 1983;ii:865–9

130. Hughs EC, Gott PS, Weinstein RC, Binggeli R. *Migraine: a diagnostic test for etiology of food sensitivity by a nutritionally supported fast and confirmed by long-term report* Ann Allergy 1985; 55:28–32

131. Smith I, Kellow AH, Hanington E. *A clinical and biochemical correlation between tyramine and migraine headache.* Headache 1970; 10:43–51

132. Perkine JE, Hartji J. *Diet and migraine: a review of the literature.* J Am Diet Assoc 1983; 83:459–63

133. Koehler SM, Glaros A. *The effect of aspartame on migraine headache.* Headache 1988; 28;10–3

134. Lipton RB, Newman LC, Solomon S. *Aspartame and headache.* N Engl J Med 1988; 318:1200–1

135. Marcus DA, Scharff L, Turk D, Gourley LM *A double blind provocative study of chocolate as a trigger of headache.* Cephalalgia 1997; 17:855–62 discussion 800

136. Becker WJ. *Use of oral contraceptives in patients with migraine.* Neurology 1999; 53 (4 Suppl 1):S19–25

137. MacGregor EA, Guillebaud J. *Migraine and stoke in young women. Authors' results suggest that all types of migraine are contraindications to oral contraceptives.* BMJ 1999; 318:1485 (letter; comment).

138. Dexter JD, Roberts J, Byer JA. *The five-hour glucose tolerance test and effect of low sucrose diet in migraine.* Headache 1978;18:91–4

139. Wilkinson CF Jr. *Recurrent migrainoid headaches associated with spontaneous hypoglycemia.* Am J Med Sci 19149; 218:209–12

140. Gallai V, Scarchielli P, Coata G, et al. *Serum and salivary magnesium levels in migraine.* Headache 1992; 32:132–35

141. Weaver K. *Magnesium and migraine.* Headache 1990; 30:168 [letter]

142. Facchinetti F, Sances G, Borella P, et al. *Magnesium prophylaxis of menstrual migraine: on intracellular migraine.* Headache 1991; 31:298–301

143. Hepinstall S, White A, et al. *Extracts of feverfew inhibit granule secretion in blood platelet polymorphonuclear leukocytes.* Lancet 1985; 1:1071–74

144. Murphy JJ, Hepinstall S, Mitchell JRA. *Randomised double-blind placebo controlled trial of feverfew in migraine prevention.* Lancet 1988; ii:189–92

145. Johnson ES, Kadam NP, et al. *Efficacy of feverfew as prophylactic treatment of migraine.* 1985; 291:569–73

146. Palevitch D, Earon G, Carasso R. *Feverfew (Tanacetum parthenium) as a prophylactic treatment for migraine:* A double-blind placebo-controlled study. Phytother Res 1997; 11:508

147. Hasselmark L, Malmgren R, Hannerz J. *Effect of a carbohydrate-rich diet, low in protein-tryptophan, in classic and common migraine.* Cephalalgia 1987; 7:87–92

148. Unge G, Malmgren R, Olsson P, et al. *Effects of dietary protein-tryptophan rstriction upon uptake by plateletsx and clinical symptoms in migraine-like headache.* Cephalalgia 1983; 3:21

149. Kimball RW, Friedman AP, Vallejo E. Effect of serotonin in migraine patients. Neurology 1960; 10:107–11

150. Sicuteri F. *The ingestion of serotonin precursors (L-F-hydroxytryptophan and L-tryptophan) improves migraine headache.* Headache 1973; 13:19–22

151. Miller JJ, Fletcher K, Kbat-Zinn. J, et.al. *Three Year follow up and clinical implications of a mindfulness meditation based stress reduction intervention in the treatment of anxiety disorders.* Gen Hosp. Psychiatry. 1995; 27:192–200

152. Bruce M et.al. *Anxiogeic.effects of caffeine in patients with anxiety disorders.* Arach Ge Psychiatry 1992; 49:867–69

153. Western PG, et.al. *Magnesium sulphate as a sedative* Am J Med Sci 1923; 165:431–33

154. Benjamin J, Levin J, Fux M, et.al. *Double-blind, placebo-controlled, crossover trial of inositol treatment for panic disorder.* Am J Psychiatry 1995; 152:1084–86.

155. Mohler H, Polc P, Cumin R, et.al. *Niacinamide is a brain constituent with benzodiazepine-like actions.* Nature 1979; 278:563–65

156. Piscopo G. *Kava Kava: Gift of the Islands.* Alt Med Rev 1997; 2:355–81[review]

157. Woelk H, Capoula S, Lehrl S, et.al. *Treatment of Patients suffering from anxiety – double blind study: Kava special extract versus benzodiazepines.* Z Allegemeied 1993; 69:271–77 [in German]

158. Whitte B, Harrer G, Kaptan T, et.al. *Treatment of depressive symptoms with a high concentration hypericum preparation.* A multi-centre placebo controlled double-blind study. Fort Schr Med. 1995; 113:404–408

159. Viola H, de Stein M L, et.al. *Apigenin a component of matricaria recutita flowers Benzidiazepine receptors – ligand with anxiolytic effects.* Planter Med 1995; 61:213–16.

160. Weiss B, Laties V G, *Enhancement of human performance by caffeine and the amphetamine (??)* Pharmacol Rev 1962; 14:1–36

161. Hollingworth HL. *The influence of caffeine on mental and motor efficiency.* Arch Phychol 1912; 20:1–66

162. Blum I, Vered Y, Graff E, et.al. *The influence of meal composition on plasma serotonin and norephinebrine concentrations.* Metabolism 1992; 41:137–40

163. Morin CM, Cuthbert J P, Schwartz S M, *Non-phamacological interventions for insomnia a mean analysis of treatment efficacy.* Am J Psychiatr 1994; 151:1172–80

164. Fuerst M L. *Insomniacs give up stress and medications.* JAMA 1983; 249:459–60

165. Haimov I, Laudon M, Zisapel N, et.al. *Sleep disorders and melatonin rhythms in elderly persons.* BMJ 1994; 309:167

166. Leathwood PD, Chauffard F, *Aqueous extract of valerian root (Valeriana officinalis) improves sleep quality in men.* Pharmacol Biochem Behav 1982; 17:65–71

167. Dressings H, Riemann D, et.al. *Insomnia — Are valerian/balm combination of equal value to benzodiazepine?* Therapiewoche 1992; 42:726–36.

168. Margetts BM, et at. *Vegetarian diet in mild hypertension:* a randomised controlled trial BNJ 1986; 293:1468–71.

169. Appel L, Moore TJ, Boarzanek E, et al. *A clinical trail of the effects of dietary patterns on blood pressure.* N Engl J Med 1997; 336:1117–24

170. Dyckner T, Wester PO. *Effect of magnesium on blood pressure* BMJ 1983; 286:1847–49

171. Narkiewicz K, Maraglino G, Biasion T, et al. *Interactive effect of cigarettes and coffee on systolic blood pressure in patients with mild essential hypertension.* J Hypertens 1995; 13:96

172. Santos MJ, Lopez-Jurado M, Llopis J, et al. *Influence of dietary supplementation with fish oils measuring plasma total cholesterol and lipoprotein cholesterol fractions in patients with coronary heart disease.* J Nutr Med 1992; 3:107–15.

173. Kromhout D, Bosschieter EB, Coulander CdL, *The inverse relation between fish consumption and 20-year mortality from coronary heart disease.* N Engl. J Med 1985; 312:1205–9

174. Thorogood M, Carter R, Benfield L, et al. *Plasma lipids and lipoprotein cholesterol concentrations in people with different diets in Britain.* Br Med J (Clin Res Ed) 1987; 295:351–53

175. Burr ML, Sweetnam PM. *Vegetarianism, dietary fiber and mortality.* Am J Clin Nutr 1982; 36:873–77

176. Resnicow K, Barone J, Engle A et al. *Diet and serum lipids in vegan vegetarians, a modest risk reduction.* J Am Dietel Assoc 1991; 91:447–53

177. Ornish D, Brown SE, Scherwitz LW, et al. *Can lifestyle changes reverse coronary heart disease.* The Lifestyle Heart Trial. Lancet 1990; 336:129–33

178. Raloff J. *Oxidised lipids: a key to heart disease?* Sci News 1985:127:278

179. Levy Y, Maor I, Presser D, Aviram M. *Consumption of eggs with meals increases the susceptibility of human plasma and low-density lipoprotein to lipid peroxidation.* Ann Nutr Met 1996; 40:243–51

180. Shekelle RB, Stamier J. *Dietary cholesterol and ischaemic heart disease.* Lancet 1989; I:79

181. Press RI, Geller J, Evans GW. *The effect of chromium picolinate on serum cholesterol and apolipoprotein fractions in human subjects.* West J. Med 1990; 152:41–45.

182. Riales R, Albrink MJ, *Effect of chromium chloride supplementation on glucose tolerance and serum lipids including high-density lipoprotein of adult men.* Am. J Clin Nutr. 1981; 34:2670–7

183. Roeback JR, Hla KM, Chambless LE, Fletcher RH. *Effects of chromium supplementation on serum high-density lipoprotein cholesterol levels in men taking beta-blockers.* Ann Intern Med 1991; 1115:917–24

184. Johanson JF, Sonnenberg A. *Constipation is not a risk factor for haemorrhoids, a case study of potential etiological agents.* Am J Gastroenterol. 1994; 89:1981–86

185. Johanson JF, Sonnenberg A. *The prevalence of hemorrhoids and chronic constipation.* Gastroenterol 1990; 98;380–86

186. Lefavi, R, Anderson R, Keith R, et al. *Efficacy of chromium supplementation in athletes: Effects on anabolism.* Int J Sport Nutr 1992; 2:1111–22

187. McCarty, MF. *The case for supplemental chromium and a survey of clinical studies with chromium picolinate.* J Appl Nutr 1991; 43:59–66

188. Cangiano C, Ceci F, Cascino A, et al. Eating *behaviour and adherence to dietary prescription obese adult subjects treated with 5–hydroxytryptophan.* Am. J Clin Nutr. 1992; 56:863–67

189. Leung A, Foster S. *Encyclopedia of common Natural Ingredients Used in Food, Drugs and Cosmetics.* 2nd Ed. New York: John Wiley & Sons, 1996, 293–94

190. Becher EW, Jakober B, Luft D, et al. *Clinical and biochemical evaluations of the algae spirulina with regard to its application in the treatment of obesity.* A double blind crossover study. Nutr Intl. 1986; 33:565–73.

191. Zackheim HS, Farber EM, Alto P – *Low Protein Diet and Psoriasis* – A Hospital Study. Arch Derm Vol 99 – May, 1969

192. Reed Suzanne, Ash M. et al. *Nutritional Treatment of Psoriasis. Does the effect of reducing liver load and increasing detoxification through dietary, lymphatic and acupressure massage techniques improve the condition of an individual suffering from psoriasis?* Research Project London, June 1993

193. Poikolainen K, Renunala, T, Karvonen J, et al. *Alcohol intake: a risk factor for psoriasis in young middle aged men?* BMJ 1990:300:780–83.

194. Monk BE, Neill SM. *Alcohol consumption and psoriasis.* Dematologicia 1986; 173:57–60

195. Ellis CN, Berberian B, Sulica VI, et al. *A double-blind evaluation of topical capsaicin in psoriasis.* J Am Acad Dermatol 1993; 29:438–42.

196. Hoffman D. *the Herbal Handbook*: A Users Guide to Medical Herbalism. Rochester, VTY: Healing Arts Press 1988, 23–24 [review]

197. Sanchez A, Reeser, JL, Lau HS, et al. *Role of sugars in human neutrophilic phagocytosis.* Clin Nutr. 1973; 26:1180–84

198. MacGregor RR. *Alcohol and immune defense.* JAMA 1986; 256:1474

199. Barone J, Herbert JR, Reddy MM. *Dietary fat and natural-killer-cell activity.* Am J Clin Nutr 1989;50:861–67

200. Axelrod DR. *Ascorbic acid and urinary pH* JAMA 1985;254:1310–11

201. Avorn J, Monane M, Gurwitz JH et al. *Reduction of bacteriuria and pyuria after ingestion of cranberry juice.* JAMA 1994; 271:751–54

202. Dignam R. Ahmed M, Denman S, et al. *The effect of cranberry juice on UTI rates in a care facility.* J Am Geriatr Soc. 1997;45:S53

203. Sobota AE. *Inhibition of bacterial adherence by cranberry juice: Potential use for the treatment of urinary tract infections.* J Urol 1984;131:1013–16

204. Bodel PT, Cotran R, Kass EH. *Cranberry juice and the antibacterial action of hippuric acid.* Clin Med 1959;54:881–88

205. Ronzio RA, *Antioxidants, nutraceuticals and functional foods.* Townsend Letter for Doctors and Patients. Oct, 1996: 34–35[review]

206. Hertog MGL, Feskens EJM, Hollman PCH, et al. *Dietary antioxidant flavonoids and risk of coronary heart disease:* the Zutphen Elderly Study Lancet 1993; 342:1007–11.

207. Grodstein F, goldman MB, Ryan L, Cramer DW. *Relation of female infertility to consumption of caffeinated beverages.* AM J Epidemiol 1993; 137:1353–60

208. Hatch EE, Brachen, MB. *Association of delayed conception with caffeine consumption* Am Epidemiol 1993; 138:1082–92

209. Wilcox A, Weinberg C, Baird D. *Caffeinated beverages and decreased fertility.* Lancet 1988 ii:1453–56

210. Howe G, Westhoff C Vessey M, Yeates D. *Effects of age, cigarette smoking and other factors in fertility: findings in a large prospective study.* BMJ 1985:290:1697–99

211. Weinberg CR, Wilcox AJ, Baird DD. *Reduced fecundability in women with prenatal exposure to cigarette smoking.* Am J Epidemiol 1989; 129:1072–78

212. Czeizel AE, Metneki J, Dudas I. *The effect of preconceptional multivitamin supplementation in fertility.* Internat J Vit Nutr Res 1996;66:55–58

213. Thiessen DD, et al. *Vitamin E and sex behaviour in mice.* Nutr Metabol 1975;18:116–119

214. Fraga CG, Motchnik PA, Shigenaga MK, et al. *Ascorbic acid protects against endogenous oxidative DNA damage in human sperm.* Proc Natl Acad Sci 1991; 88:11003–6

215. Dawson EB, Harris WA, McGanity WJ. *Effect of ascorbic acid on sperm fertility.* Fed Proc 1983;42:531 [abstr 31403]

216. Hunt CD, Johnson PE, Herbel JoL, Mullen LK. *Effects of dietary zinc depletion on seminal and zinc loss, serum testerone concentrations, and sperm morphology in young men.* Am Nutr 1992; 56:148–57

217. Netter A, Hartoma R, Nahoul K. *Effect of zinc administration on plasma testosterone, dihydrotestosterone and sperm count.* Arch Androl 1981; 7:69–73

218. Marmar JL et al. *Semen zinc levels in infertile and postvasectomy patients and patients with prostatitis.* Fertil Steril 1975;26:1057–63

219. Galeao R. *La dysmenorrhee, syndrome multiforme.* Gynecologie 1974;25:125 [in French]

220. Harel Z, Biro FM, Kottenhahn RK, Rosenthal SL. *Supplementation with omega-3 polyunsaturated fatty acids in the management of dysmenorrhoea in adolescents.* Am J Obstet Gynecol 1996; 174:1335–38

221. Reiter WJ, Pycha A, Schatzl G et al. *Dehydroepindrosterone in the treatment of erectile dysfunction: a prospective, double blind randomized, placebo-controlled study.* Urology 1999; 53:590–95

222. Sohn M, Sikora R. *Ginkgo biloba extract for antidepressant-induced sexual dysfunction.* J Sex Educ 1991; 17:53–61.

223. Kunelius P, Hakkinen J, Lukkarinen O. *Is high-dose yohimbine hydrochlorine effective in the treatment of mixed-type impotence? A prospective, randomized controlled double-blind cross over study* Urol 1997; 49:441–44

224. Mann K, Klingler T, Noe S, et al. *Effect of yohimbine on sexual experiences and nocturnal tumescence and rigidity in erectile dysfunction.* Arch Sex Behav 1996; 25:1–16

225. Rossignol AM Bonniander H. *Prevalence and severity of the premenstrual syndrome. Effects of foods and beverages that are sweet or high in sugar content.* J Reprod Med 1991; 36:131–3.

226. Rossignol AM. *Caffeine-containing beverages and premenstrual syndrome in young women.* Public Health 1985; 75(11): 1335–37.

227. Rossignol AM. Bonniander H. *Caffeine-containing beverages total fluid consumption and premenstrual syndrome.* Am J Public Health 1990; 80: 1106–10.

228. Prior JC, Vigna Y, Sciarretta D, et al. *Conditioning exercise decreases premenstrual symptoms. A prospective, controlled 6-month trial.* Fertil Steril 1987;47(3):402–408

229. McFayden IJ, Forest AP et al. *Cyclical breast pain – some observations and the difficulties of treatment.* Br J Clin Pract 1992; 46:161–64

230. Bohnert KJ, Hahn G. *Phytotherpay in gynecology and obstretics — Vitex Agnes Castus.* Erfahrungsheikunde 1990; 39:494–502

231. Lauritzen C, Reuter HD, Repges R, et al. Treatment of premenstrual tension syndrome with Vitex Agnes Castus. Controlled, double blind study versus pyridoxine. Phytomedicine 1997; 4:183–86

232. Genton C, Frie PC, Pecoud A. *Value of oral provocation tests to aspirin and food additives in routine investigation of asthma and chronic urticaria.* J Asthma 1985;76:40–45

233. Townes SJ, Mellis *CM. Role of acetyl salicylic acid and sodium metabisulfite inchronic child asthma.* Pediatr 1984; 73:631–37

234. Rowe AH, Young EJ. *Bronchial asthma due to food allergy alone in ninety-five patients.* J Asthma 1959; 169:1158

235. Weir MR et al. *Depression of vitamin B6 levels due to theophyline.* Ann Allergy 1990; 65:52–62

236. Reynolds RD, Natta CL. *Depressed plasma pyridoxal phosphate concentrations in adult asthmatics.* Am J Clin Nutr 1985; 41: 684–88

237. Zuskin E et al, *Byssinosis and airway responses due to exposure to textile dust.* Lung 1976; 154:17–24

238. Ruskin SL *Sodium ascorbate in the treatment of allergic disturbances. The role of adrenal cortical hormone-sodium-vitamin C.* Am J Dig Dis 1947;14:302–306

239. Welton AF, Tobias LD, Fiedler-Nagy C, et al. *Effect of flavonoids on arachidonic acid metabolism.* Prog Clin Biol Res 1986; 213:231–42

240. Ascherio A, Willett WC. *Health effects of trans fatty acids.* Am J Clin Nutr 1997; 66(suppl):1006S-10S[review]

241. Ornish D, Brown SE, Scherwitz LW, et al. *Can lifestyle changes reverse coronary heart disease.* Lancet 1990; 336: 129–33.

242. Olson BH, Anderson SM Becker MP, et al. *Psyllium-enriched cereals lower blood total cholesterol and LDL cholesterol, but not HDL cholesterol, in hypercholesterolemic adults.* A meta analysis. J Nutr 1997; 127: 1973–80.

243. Braquet O, Touqui L, Shen TS, Vargaftig BB, *Perspectives in platelet activating factor* Pharmacol Rev 1987;39:97–210

244. Blumenthal M, Busse WR, Goldberg A, et.al, Eds. *The Completely German Commission Monographs: Therapeutic Guide to Herbal Medicines* Austin, TX: American Botanical Boston: Integrative Medicine Communications 1998, 149

245. Kreysel HW, Nissen HP, Enghofer E. *A possible role of lysosomal enzymes in the pathogenic varicosis and the reduction in their serum activity by Venostasin* Vasa 1983;12:377–82

246. Levy JA,Ibrahim AB, Shirai T, et al. *Dietary fat affects immune response, production of ant factors, and immune complex disease in NZP/NZW mice.* Proc Natl Acad Sci 1982;79:1974

247. Darlington LG, Ramsey NW *Diets for rheumatoid arthritis.* Lancet 1991;338:1209 [letter]

248. Scherak O, Kolarz G. *Vitamin E and rheumatoid arthritis.* Arthrit Rheum 1991;34:1205–1210[letter]

249. General Practitioner Research Group. *Calcium pantothenate in arthritic conditions* Practit 1980; 224:208–211

250. DiSilvestro RA, Marten J, Skeham M. *Effects of copper supplementation on ceruloplasmin copper-zinc superoxide dismutase in free-living rheumatoid arthritis patients.* J Am Coll Nutr 1992;11:177–80

251. Medical News. *Copper boosts activity of anti-inflammatory drugs.* JAMA 1974; 229:1268

252. Belch JJF, Snsell D, Madhok R, et al. *Effects of altering dietary essential fatty acids on requirements for non-steroidal anti-inflammatory drugs.* Brit J Rheumatol 1991;30:370–72

253. Hemila H. *Does Vitamin C alleviate the symptoms of the common cold? A review of current evidence* Scand J Infect Dis 1994;26:1–6

254. Macknin ML. *Zinc lozenges for the common cold.* Cleveland Clin J Med 1999;66:27–32[review]

255. Schulz V, Hansel R, Tyler VE. *Rational Phytotherapy*, 3rd ed. Berlin, Germany; Springer Verlag 1998; 146–47

256. Sanchez A, Resser JL, Lau HS, et al. *Role of sugars in human neutrophilic phagocytosis.* Clin Nutr 1973; 26:1180–84

257. Hunt C, Chakravorty NK, Annan G et.al. *The clinical effects of vitamin C supplementation in elderly hospitalised patients with acute respiratory infections.* Int J Vitam Nutr Res 1994; 64:2

258. Grassi C, Morandini GC. *A controlled trial of intermittent oral acetylcysteine in the long-term treatment of chronic bronchitis.* Eur J Clin Pharmacol 1976; 9:393–96.

259. Boman G, Backer U, Larsson, S et al *Oral acetylcysteine reduces exacerbation rate in chronic bronchitis: report of a trial organized by the Swedish Society for Pulmonary Diseases* Eur J Dis 1983; 64:405–15

260. Riise GC, Larsson S, Larsson P, et al. *The intrabronchial microbial flora in chronic bronchitis patients: a target for N-acetylcysteine therapy?* Eur Respir J 1994; 7:94–101

261. Blunenthal M, Busse WR, Goldberg A. et al. *The complete German Commission E Mono Therapeutic Guide to Herbal Medicines.* Austin, Texas: American Botanical Council, 1998.

262. Bullock C. *Chronic infectious sinusitis linked to allergies.* Med Trib 1995;Dec 7:1

263. Clemetson CA. *Histamine and ascorbic acid in human blood.* J Nutr 1980; 110:662–68

264. Taub SJ *The use of bromelains in sinusitis: a double-blind evaluation.* EENT Monthly 1999 (3):361–65

265. Schulz V, Hansel R, Tyler VE. *Rational Phytotherapy* 3rd ed. Berllin, Germany: Springer Verlag 1998; 146–47

266. Manku MS, Horrobin DF, Morse NL et al. *Essential fatty acids in the plasma phospholipids of patients with atopic eczema.* Br J Dermatol 1984;110:643–48

267. Bjorneboe A, Soyland E,Bjorneboe G-EA, et al. *Effect of dietary supplementation with eicosapentaenoic acid in the treatment of atopic dermatitis.* Br J Dermatol 1987; 117:463–69

268. Threlkeld DS, et al. *Hormones, Antidiabetic Agents, Insulin. In Facts and Comparisons Drug Information.* St Louis MO. Facts and Comparisons Oct, 1997, 129f-129j.

269. Ivasson T, Spetz AC, Hammr M. *Physical exercise and vasomotor symptoms in postmenopausal women.* Mauritas 1998 29:139–46

270. Hammar M, Berg G, Lindgren R. *Does physical exercise influence the frequency of postmenopausal hot flushes?* Acta Obstet Gynecol Scand. 1990; 69:409–12.

271. Slaven L, Lee C. *Mood and symptom reporting among middle-aged women: the relationship between menopausal status, hormone replacement therapy, and exercise participation.* Healt Psychol 1997; 16:203–8.

272. Perloff WH. *Treatment of the menopause.* Am J Obstet Gynecol 1949;58:684–94

273. Gozan HA. *The use of vitamin E in treatment of the menopause.* NY State J Med 1952; 52:1289

274. Christy CJ. *Vitamin E in menopause: Preliminary report of experimental and clinical study* Obstet Gynecol 1945; 50:84

275. Finkler RS. *The effect of vitamin E in the menopause.* J clin Endocrin Metab 1949; 9:8

276. Rubenstein BB. *Vitamin E diminishes the vasomotor symptoms of menopause.* Fed Proc 1948; 7:106[abstract]

277. Knight DC, Eden JA. A review of the clinical effects of phytoestrogens. Obstet Gynecol 1996;87:897–904 [review]

278. Duker EM. *Effects of extracts from Cimicifuga racemosa on gonadotropin release in menopausal women and ovariectomized rats.* Planta Med 1991; 57:420–24

279. Lieberman S. *A review of the effectiveness of Cimicifuga racemost (black cohosh) for the symptoms of menopause.* J Women's Health 1998; 7:525–29.

280. Duke JA. *CRC Handbook of Medicinal Herbs.* Boca Raton, FL: CRC Press, 1985, 420–425 [review]

281. Bach D, Eleling L. *Long-term drug treatment of benign prostatic hyperplasia – results of a prospective 3-year multicenter study using Sabal extract* IDS 89. Phytomedicine 1996; 3:105 (originally published in Urologe (b) 1995;35:178–83)

282. Andro MC, Riffaud JP. *Pygeum africanum extract for the treatment of patients with benign hyperplasia. A systematic review of 25 years of published experience.* Curr Ther Res 1995;56:817

283. Damrau F. *Benign prostatic hypertrophy; amino acid therapy for symptomatic relief.* J Am Soc 1962; 10;426–30.

284. Fahim, M., Fahim Z, Der, R and Marman J. *Zinc treatment for the reduction of hyperplasia of the prostate.* Fed Proc 35:361,1976

285. Bock SA, Lee W-Y, Remigio LK, May DC. *Studies of hypersensitivity reactions to foods in adults and children.* J Allerg Clin Immunol 1978; 62:327–34

286. O'Shea JA, Porter SF. J *Learning Disabilities* 1981; 14(4):189–91

287. Salzman LK. *Allergy testing, psychological assessment and dietary treatment of the hypersensitive child syndrome.* Med J Australia 1976; Aug 14:248–51

288. Crook WG *Food and chemical allergies: relationship to behaviour.* J Applied Nutr 1983;3(1):47–53

289. *Allergies may led to minimal brain dysfunction in children* JAMA 1970;212(1):33–34

290. Breneman JC. *Allergy elimination diet as the most effective gallbladder diet.* Ann Allergy 1968; 26:83.

291. Cox IM, Campbell MJ, Dowson D. *Red blood cell magnesium and chronic fatigue syndrome.* Lancet 1991; 340:426

292. Kuratsune H, Yamaguti K, Takahashi M, et al. *Acylcarnitine deficiency in chronic fatigue syndrome* Clin Infect Dis 1994; 18(suppl 1) S62–67

293. Muller, DPR, *Vitamin E and neurological function.* Redox Rep 1:239–45, 1995

294. Childers NF *A relationship of arthritis to the solanaceae (nightshades)* J Internat Acad Pre 1982; Nov: 31–37

295. Childers NF, Margoles MC. *An apparent relationship of nightshades (Solanaceae) to arthritis* J Orthop Med Surg 1993; 14:227–31.

296. Schumacher HR. Osteoarthritis: *The clinical picture, pathogenesis, and management with a new therapeutic agent, S-adenosylmethionine.* Am J Med 1987; 83(suppl 5A): 48–54.

297. Harmand MF, Vilamitjana J, Maloche E,et al. *Effects of S-adenosylmethionine on human articular chondrocyte differentiation. An in vitro study.* Am J Med 1987; 83(suppl 5A) 48–54.

298. Safayhi H, Mach T, Saieraj J, etal. *Boswellic acids: Novel specific, nonredox inhibitors of lipoxygenase* J Pharmacol Exp Ther 1992; 261:1143–46.

Further Reading

Balancing Hormones Naturally, Kate Neil & Patrick Holford, Piatkus (1998)

Optimum Nutrition Bible, Patrick Holford, Piatkus (1997)

What Your Doctor Didn't Tell You About Menopause Dr. John Lee, Warner Books (1996)

Fats that Heal, Fats That Kill, Udo Erasmus, Alive Books (1970)

The Waterfall Diet Linda Lazarides Piatkus, ISBN 0–7499–2025–4

Appendix 1

RECOMMENDED SUPPLEMENT COMPANIES

SOLGAR VITAMINS

(available from all good health food stores)
For B12 nuggets (sublingual B12)
VM75 – a good all-round multivitamin and mineral supplement
Saw Palmetto, Don Quai, and all other Herbal remedies recommended in this book

BIOCARE

Lakeside Centre
180 Lifford Lane
Kings Norton,
Birmingham, B30 3NU
Technical Team — 0121 433 8720
for Replete Probiotics — powdered probiotics to be made into a drink

HEALTH PLUS LIMITED

Dolphin House,
30 Lushington Road
Eastbourne,
East Sussex BN21 4LL
Tel 01323 737374
For Metabolic Pack, Pregnancy Pack, Menopause Pack, Teenage Pack & Joint Pack

Higher Nature Limited

The Nutrition Centre,
Burwash Common,
East Sussex TN19 7LX
Tel: 01435 882880
For Starflower, Pro-Gest cream and oil from Mexican Yam and Es-Gen cream

ONC – Optimum Nutrition Company

P O BOX 88
Bracknell
RG12 1JF
01344 301344
(Practioner only service)
For Udo's Choice – A liquid blend of essential fatty acids.
Nutri Hair, and a wide range of quality products)

Useful Addresses

DIAGNOSTIC TESTING FACILITIES:

BIOLAB MEDICAL UNIT

9 Weymouth Street,
London, W1N 3FF
020 7636 5959
Referral from a GP required via nutrition consultant.

DOCTORS LABORATORY PLC

58 Wimpole Street
London
W1M 7DE
071 224 1001
No appointment necessary —
for many endocrine tests: Impotence, Menopausal, Thyroid, HRT, female and male
infertility, prostate, anaemia, and allergy screens

HEALTH INTERLINK – DIAGNOSTIC LABORATORY SERVICE

Redbourn,
Hertfordshire
AL3 7JX
01582 794094

Appendix II

ANSWERS TO SELF-TESTS

Self Test 1 – Carbohydrates.

Q1.   What is the main function of carbohydrates?

A1.   Carbohydrates are our primary source of energy.

Q2.   What is the main difference between mono-saccahrides and polysaccahrides?

A2.   The main difference between mono-saccarides and polysaccharides are that mono-saccarides water-soluble. This means they are readily absorbed into the body through the stomach giving a burst of energy. Polysaccharides, on the other hand, need digesting through the small intestine, and give a more steady energy burst for a longer period of time.

Q3.   Give 5 reasons why fiber is important in the diet

A3.   Lowers harmful cholesterol levels. (Soluble)
Reduces the risk of cardiovascular disease. (Soluble)
Eases bowel movements by making stools slippery. (Soluble)
Provides food for beneficial bacteria in the intestines. (Soluble)
Help against weight gain, colon cancer and gallstones. (Insoluble)

Q4.   What are enzymes?

A4.   They are protein catalysts. Enzymes are energised protein molecules that perform specific biochemical reactions vital for life.

Q5.   Name the enzyme needed for the breakdown of carbohydrates in the body

A5.   Amylase

Self Test 2 – Proteins

Q1.   How many essential amino acids are there?

A1.   There are 8 Essential amino acids. These are Isoleucine, Leucine, Lysine, Methionine, Phenylalanine, Threonine, Tryptophan, and

Valine. In addition are 2 amino acids that are regarded essential in children, being Arginine and Histidine.

Q2. What are the main functions of protein?
A2. For the growth and repair of body tissues and production of enzymes.

Q3. What is a 'limiting' amino acid?
A3. A limiting amino acid is an amino acid that is present in relatively small amounts and below the recommended essential amino acid requirements.

Q4. What 4 particular nutrients are needed by the liver to convert the essential amino acids to other amino acids?
A4. Vitamins A, B6, Vitamin K and B12 are the important nutrients needed to convert and rebuild amino acids.

Q5. Which particular essential amino acid is often low in vegetarian diets and what foods can this be found in?
A5. Lysine is often low in vegetarian diets.

Self Test 3 – Fats

Q1. What are the three main divisions of fats?
A1. Saturated fats, mono-unsaturated fats and poly-unsaturated fats.

Q2. What are the main functions of fats?
A2. Fats provide a highly concentrated source of energy, which can be stored and used instead of carbohydrates when necessary. Fats provide us with insulation and protect delicate body organs. Fats also produce highly active biological substances that are vital for the normal working of the body. These substances are known as prostaglandins.

Q3. What are prostaglandins?
A3. Prostaglandins are hormone like substances which are very short lived and have important functions in the body They help keep the blood thin, they have anti-inflammatory influences on the joints, they prevent fluid retention, they help lower blood pressure and help insulin work efficiently.

Q4. How can fibre help lower cholesterol levels

A4. Soluble fibre takes up bile acids, cholesterol and toxins and carries them out of the body

Q5. What are the four functions of cholesterol?

A5. It is a constituent of cell membranes.

It is a precursor of bile acids.

It is a precursor of steroid hormones.

Vitamin D, the sunshine vitamin, also comes from cholesterol.

Self Test 4 – Supplements

Q1. Vitamins are divided into two main divisions. What are they?

A1. The water-soluble vitamins of the B complex group and vitamin C and the fat-soluble vitamins A, D, E and K.

Q2. What do the initials SONA stand for and when should we use them?

A2. SONA – Suggested Optimal Nutritional Allowance – are the levels of nutrients that are more likely to be used to maintain optimum health.

Q3. An excess of copper in the body may result in a deficiency of which mineral?

A3. Zinc

Q4. What is Co-Q-10 and what is its function?

A4. Co-Q-10, is a component of every living cell, and its function is to improve the cell's ability to use oxygen,

Q5. What are the antioxidants, and what is their main function?

A5. The antioxidants are the vitamins A, C and E and the mineral Selenium. Their main function is to protect body cells against free radicals.

Self Test 5 – Herbal Remedies

Q1. What is the main function of herbs?

A1. The main functions of herbs are for food, medicine, scent, and flavour.

Q2.   Which herb has anti-histamine, antioxidant and anti-inflam-matory properties and is usually recommended for allergies?

A2.   Quercetin

Q3.   Which herb has anti-depressant, anti-bacterial, and sedative properties and is usually recommended for mild depression?

A3.   St. John's Wort

Q4.   What important difference must you remember between the herbs Vitex (Agnus Castus) and Black Cohosh?

A4.   Vitex and black cohosh have *opposite* actions Use black cohosh for low estrogen levels (30% of clients) and vitex for high estrogen (70% of clients)

Q5.   If a client had poor circulation, especially to their hands and feet, what herb might you consider?

A5.   Ginkgo Biloba

Self Test 5 – Super Foods

Q1.   What superfood would you consider for a vegan or strict vegetarian?

A1.   The algae group of superfoods — Spirulina, Chlorella and Blue-Green Algae.

Q2.   Honey can be described as a prebiotic. What are prebiotics, and what other foods come into this category?

A2.   Prebiotics stimulates the activity of the body's own existing good bacteria. Other foods include chicory, artichoke, garlic, onion, leek, asparagus, peaches and bananas.

Q3.   Which superfood is anti-bacterial, anti-viral, and heals stomach ulcers?

A3.   Cabbage

Q4.   Which of the superfoods his anti-viral properties, and benefits respiratory tract infections?

A4.   Licqurice

Q5. What are the main functions of Bee Pollen?

A5. Bee pollen enhances fertility, it is an antioxidant, it enhances vitality, is a natural tonic, strengthens the immune system, is natural anti-histamine, regulates blood pressure, and assists weight loss, colitis and constipation.

Q6. Unlike blue-green algae, spirulina and chlorophyll, mushrooms lack chlorophyll. Where do these medicinal mushrooms obtain their healing properties?

A6. Medicinal mushrooms absorb nutrients from the surrounding medium such as soil, decaying wood and other forest waste material.

VTCT – Vocational Training Charitable Trust

VTCT started life in 1962 providing the first high level National Qualifications in Beauty Therapy. Since then it has expanded to offer Hairdressing, Customer Service, Key Skills and other qualifications approved by QCA (Qualifications and Curriculum Authority) and SQA (Scottish Qualifications Authority) as well as being the market leader in Beauty Therapy, Fitness, Sports and Holistic Therapies. The qualifications of VTCT are available at over 350 centers around the country. These centers are mostly Colleges of Further Education, the remainder being made up of private colleges and schools.

FHT – Federation of Holistic Therapists

The Federation of Holistic Therapists is the largest professional association for therapists in the UK. They are a non-profit making organisation seeking to represent their members at national level. The FHT publishes the Code of Practice for Hygiene in Salons and Clinics which is the standard guideline for their industry, and all members must abide by their Code of Ethics.

The Federation is made up of five societies:-

IFHB   –   International Federation of Health & Beauty Therapists
ICHT   –   International Council of Holistic Therapists
HFST   –   International Council of Health, Fitness & Sports Therapists
ATL   –   Association of Therapy Lecturers
HBEL –   Health & Beauty Employers Federation

Health & Beauty Enterprises

Established in 1989 Health and Beauty Enterprises, offers comprehensive training in vocational and complementary therapies, and offer courses accredited by VTCT. The Home Study Diploma course in Nutrition, written by Suzanne Reed-Le Quesne, will be of interest to anyone with an interest in food and its influence of our health and is available from the web-site. H&BE also teach the holistic disciplines of Aromatherapy, Indian Head Massage, Reflexology, and Reiki.

For a full schedule of courses and workshops visit http://www.suzanne-reed.com or call +44(0)1584 861560

HOME STUDY DIPLOMA COURSE IN NUTRITION
Accredited by Vocational Awards International

Aim: To enable the student to communicate effectively with their clients on nutrition and supplement requirements and to be able to organise for them a balanced diet taking into account their individual requirements.

By the end of the course you will have a workable knowledge of the following: -

Course Content:
M74 — Support Employment Standards
Assignment covering hygiene and safety in the workplace, confidentiality, and how to treat clients professionally. Written questions as assignment

M61 – Provide Advice on Nutrition

The Digestive System and The Urinary System
Knowledge of and important sources of Proteins, Fats, Carbohydrates, Vitamins & Minerals
Nutritional Deficiencies
Absorption of nutrients and their utilisation in the body
Food energy values (Kcals/Kjoules)(Food Groups)
Important sources and functions of fibre
The requirements/benefits of a balanced diet
Published dietary norms, including the National Food Guide, National guidelines
Body Mass index and its application
Fluid balance in the body, brief knowledge of hormonal factors affecting this and how it can be affected by diet.
Effects of dietary intake on adipose tissue
Effects of exercise in utilising food intake
Effect of restrictive diet, appetite suppressant pills, health food myths, dieter's food etc.
Consultation techniques – how to assess clients for deficiencies
Case Studies provided – Doreen, David and Richard.

Additional Information — All qualifications are performance related — competence based on skills knowledge, understanding, ability in application. Evaluation is by continuous assessment therefore frequent tests will be give, as will some written essays, small assignments projects etc. as homework.

Length of course — Home study course consisting of 8 Modules — You decide how long you wish to take. Recommended 1 module per month. Recommended reading list given for background information and knowledge to know the subject thoroughly.

Start whenever you want to; study when you want to; study where you want to.

INDEX